Saving Sandy

Sandy tells her story as understood by the heart of Diana.

Diana B. Mahoney

A Note by the Author

This book is dedicated to all of those wonderful friends who followed Sandy's Facebook page throughout her life with us. Their steadfast and loving support helped give Sandy the very best life could offer, which she so richly deserved. Their cards, emails, comments and messages were a daily inspiration, and we felt as if we had gained a whole world of friends. At its highest point, Sandy had over 16,000 followers on Facebook. Many of you, like Rex, Nancy and Michelle and Diana, Sallie, Suzi, Rocky, Elizabeth, Robin, Erica, Glenda, Janice, Mamy, Sue, MaryAnn, Sandy, Rose, Fiona, Agnes, Charles, Mary, and on and on, thousands of you have kept in touch, and this book would not be happening without your encouragement and persistence. We know your names by recognition and are forever humbled.

We also owe a debt of gratitude to Dr. Ruth West, owner of Karma K9 Mobile Acupuncture of Wake County, North Carolina. Dr. Ruth's compassion, gentle nature and skills allowed Sandy much comfort on the days when she needed it so much. Her visits to us were always welcome, and we became true believers in the practice of acupuncture to relieve Sandy's tension, anxiety, and discomfort.

In addition, the answer from my husband, "Well, we have to save her," was life-changing. He never wavered in the work to be done, the patience required, and the dedication to making Sandy's life wonderful. He is a good soul who loves animals deeply, and Sandy was lucky to have him as her Dad. Special thanks to him who shared this journey, who put up with my late hours so I could keep her Facebook Family up to date and who gave his heart to this beautiful dog.

Acknowledgments

At the beginning of Saving Sandy, a wonderful woman became one of Sandy's most loyal followers. Through the years that have passed, Jo Ann McKahan Gilbert has stayed in touch and, early on, took a special interest in the possibility of a book. She offered her assistance in editing this book, and I am eternally grateful for her talents and willingness to undertake this part of publishing. Jo is a former reporter/editor for the Panhandle Press, the Columbiana Ledger, a former reporter for The Vindicator and Morning Journal and currently a freelance journalist. I have great appreciation and admiration for her talents and a friendship that will last forever.

To my Amazon publishing team, I am blessed with their work and support in making this book a reality. My work with them was cohesive and thorough, and their knowledge was a guiding light.

About the Author

Diana Blackburn Mahoney is a native Virginian and resides in Midlothian, Virginia, with her husband, Michael. She grew up in Waynesboro, Virginia, in the heart of the Shenandoah Valley. Diana and Michael met as students at the University of Richmond, where Diana majored in journalism, psychology, and secondary education and later did work on her Master's degree in psychology. Her work career was spent with Procter and Gamble, Johnson and Johnson and Altria. Her husband, Michael, is a former owner of several jewelry retail stores and has been CFO of two corporations. Prior to his working career, he played in the NFL. They are both now retired.

They live with their German Shepherd/Huskie mix and their black Labrador Retriever, both of whom they adopted from rescues. Juniper was adopted as a pup from Shenandoah Shepherd Rescue, and Rocky was adopted from Lab Rescue of Virginia. Their cat, Lulu, was also rescued from Tabby and Pup in Midlothian, VA.

Diana volunteers with three rescue organizations; Best Friends of Kanab, Utah, Doobert East Coast Animal Transport, and Shenandoah Shepherd Rescue.

Prologue

In preparation for the 2014 Christmas season, there was the usual discussion with family members about the exchange of gifts. Our family is small in number and, traditionally, giving amongst us had always been heartfelt but extravagant in comparison to the lives we lived as children. Our post-WWII parents had always seen to the needs of our family, and the wants were kept in check by very slim sums in the checking accounts. But that said, we always had pets. We had cats and kittens, and puppies and dogs. We had turtles and hamsters, goldfish, and a garter snake. We loved them with all of our hearts and wept over each one when they made the change from now into forever.

Well, back to the exchange of gifts. No one seemed particularly responsive to requests for lists, and we began the realization that we could make a difference by doing something differently. We decided each family member could choose a charity or foundation, and a gift would be made in their honor to the charity of their choice.

Among their choices were non-profit organizations like Corolla Wild Horse Foundation, Best Friends Animal Sanctuary and others. My sister and her husband were dedicated owners of two dearly loved German Shepherd dogs, Maggie and Boz, so one of the gifts included a donation to Southeast German Shepherd Rescue in honor of my brother-in-law. Obtaining the certificate and donating the gift was done online, and thus my name and information was given to them. I don't recall if I checked any box saying I'd be willing to adopt or foster a dog.

My husband and I are "Mom" and "Dad" to four rescued four-legged children. Tipper; a tortoise shorthair kitten of a feral cat who landed in my sister's yard, and Lulu; a mostly Maine Coon kitten of a rescued feral mom, make up the cat part of the family. Annie, a probable mix of golden retriever and border collie, came in 2006 after being found as a six-week-old pup abandoned in the barn where our daughter's horse was stabled. Buddy, a tri-colored cocker spaniel mix, traveled to the east coast as a result of my visit to Best Friends Animal Sanctuary to volunteer in Kanab, Utah at the Sanctuary. I traveled to Best Friends with my dear college friend, Dr. Joan DaVanzo, to volunteer as a result of learning about them rescuing the Vicktory Dogs. Their story had reached deeply into my heart. I am a Virginian and was living in the city where Michael Vick was tried and convicted for heinous crimes against dogs. Volunteers at the sanctuary are encouraged to take a pet home for an overnight stay in their lodging. All the hotels, motels, and cottages welcome these pets, and one night while there, we took a precious lonely cocker mix for an overnight. Once Buddy did a sleepover with us, there was no way Joan was going to leave him there. The next thing I knew, she had paid his airfare, and I was on the way to Dulles Airport to pick him up.

Best Friends Animal Sanctuary changed my life. It was the deepest, most profound spiritual experience I have ever had. It is living witness to the intertwined spirits of living and loving and giving and receiving. It is the heart of goodness and mercy here on this small planet we call Earth. I am forever blessed by the purpose I found in this place, by the people who sacrificed to make this place and for helping to continue the mission of Best Friends Animal Sanctuary.

I thank them for the gift they gave to me. I thank my husband, Michael, for his understanding and never-ending commitment to sharing my purpose and for knowing the gift of loving an animal.

I have enormous gratitude for the Facebook Family I found when I established a page called Saving Sandy, thus the title of this book. They, in no small part, stood by us when Sandy was so fragile, cheered her (and us) every day and made things possible for Sandy, which we could never have done without them. Sandy's family grew to over 16,000 who followed her. The prayers and healing energies sent her way worked miracles. This family walked through saving this German Shepherd and is proof positive that, as humans, we can form loving relationships without ever meeting face to face. In a world of so much information and access to immediate communication, these relationships continue to this day.

The Soul of Sandy

We rescued a dog.

She rescued us.

We fed her body.

She fed our souls.

We encouraged her.

She showed us courage.

We gave her a home.

She gave us purpose.

We cared for her needs.

She opened our hearts.

We were her legs.

She was our guardian.

We shared her with the world.

She shared her trust with us.

We gave her back to God to be healed.

She lives to walk and run.

We can only strive to be as loving and forgiving as she.

She set the example.

It is for us to follow.

"If a man aspires towards a righteous life, his first act of abstinence
is from injury to animals."

~Albert Einstein

Allow Me to Introduce Myself

January 2016

My name is Sandy. I am a 10-year-old German Shepherd and I really don't know why I am still alive. For so many years I hoped things would get better, and I just wanted to have someone pet me and not abuse me. Then, I realized I wasn't going to be loved, and I would stand outside in the biting rain and bone-chilling cold and smothering heat and terrifying storms until a human being would see me and realize how badly I needed help.

No one knows how long I was hungry and neglected, but somehow a policeman came along, and I finally got taken to a shelter, after what was thought to be about 10 years of people being awful to me. But .... then I realized that no one would want me at my age looking and smelling like I did. You see, I had mange all over my body, I should have weighed 85 to 95 pounds, but I only weighed 52 pounds, and my ears were so infected that I smelled. So I had been on death row for about 6 weeks, which is longer than most of my friends at the shelter. Every morning more of them would be led away and never come back. A kind shelter volunteer named Sandy worked hard every day to find someone to save me.

Then a miracle happened. Southeast German Shepherd Rescue put me on their list to be saved, and I got a bath and waited, but no one came. The shelter told Southeast German Shepherd that I would cross the rainbow bridge on January 5th, 2016. I overheard the caregivers talking and saying a loving lady named Lorraine had bought me two more days of life. I was so weak I couldn't stand up and I was really tired of my burning itching skin. But most of all, I just didn't want to be hungry ever again. I tried to show all of the people who came to care for me what a really nice girl I am, and if someone could help me

9

get well I'd be a loving companion. Sandra thought I was pretty special, and she must have worked hard with Lorraine because all of a sudden I had to be bathed and disinfected and they tried to clean the pus out of my ears, but it hurt me so badly. The next thing I knew was that a kind sweet lady and a nice man came in to get me and she cried and cried when she looked at me. I didn't have a mirror so I didn't know how bad I looked, but I know how badly I felt. They put me in the car and took me to a doctor's office. I couldn't stand up on the floor because my legs would not hold me and because my nails had gotten so long they curled under. They tried to trim my nails at the shelter, but they had gotten too long to cut them very short and would bleed if trimmed short enough for me to walk on them.

A nice lady and man came into the examining room and were so soft and gentle with me. I wondered if someone was going to put me back in the cold and rain and starve me because I knew it wouldn't be long before I died if they did. But, the new people put me in their car on a big soft thing they called "your bed" and brought me to their house. I had to go to the park first with my new foster dad, so my new foster mom could bring some new friends to meet me. Their names are Annie and Buddy, and they were very nice to me. It turns out that they are my new foster family, and they actually wanted me to come inside their house. They helped me get out of the car and we went inside where they put that soft thing "your bed" on the floor. Then it was a miracle! They gave me a big bowl of food and all the nice things made me really uneasy. But I hurt so badly and was so hungry that even though I was starving and tired I was a little out of it. I couldn't believe the food and the "your bed".

Notes from the Author

My name is Diana, and my husband is Michael. On a Tuesday evening in January 2016, I got the phone call that began the end to Sandy's abuse and neglect. We met the rescue at the veterinary office, and although I thought I was prepared to see this German Shepherd named Sandy, I was panic-stricken when we entered the exam room. My heart broke and I felt so helpless because this girl was in such horrible condition. I didn't know if our love could heal her, if we had the skill to nurse her, or if she would live long enough to get through the night, but I knew we were her only chance. With faith and hope, we barreled ahead with an overwhelming knowledge of the commitment we were making and the determination to make at least her last day or days filled with comfort and love.

Sandy joined our family in January 2016.

Today we reside in the Midlothian Virginia area along with Lulu, who is still with us, Juniper, and Rocky. We have mourned over the loss of so many of our pets; Sandy, Buddy, Annie, Cash, Tipper, Katie, Simone, Sunshine, Will, Ladybug, Morris, and Noodle. Their lives made ours better. We are happy to share this wonderful story told in the voice of Sandy, who reached over 16,000 people through her media page.

The Call

"When the Man waked up he said 'What is the wild dog doing here?' And the Woman said 'His name is not Wild Dog anymore but the First Friend because he will be your friend for always, and always and always.'"

~ Rudyard Kipling from The Jungle Book

<u>2016</u>

Unexpected calls with no caller ID rarely get answered by me on my cell phone. I was leaving rehearsal with the North Carolina Master Chorale when my phone rang. For some reason only known by the universe, I answered. The caller identified herself as a representative from Southeast German Shepherd Rescue.

The call came one evening in January 2016 about a German Shepherd named Sandy, who was on the kill list for Friday, January 15. I was told that the dog was in terrible shape and was begged by the caller to foster this helpless dog. I was at a loss for words, my mind was racing, and my questions came so fast that I could not even ask them. All I could say was that I was on my way to a rehearsal, and I needed to speak with my husband about it. I asked if she could call back in the morning.

After a thoughtful drive home following rehearsal, I decided to rely on the more practical judgment of my husband. I talked it over with Michael, whose response was simply, "Well, we have to take her. We can't just let her die." I immediately went online, as instructed, and filled out the foster parent form. I would receive a call the next morning.

Sure enough, the call came, and our paperwork and approval had been expedited. The lovely lady from Southeast German Shepherd Rescue came to our home to make sure we were fit foster parents. After the home visit, we went to shop for an orthopedic dog bed. I received pictures of the dog, and they were horrifying. She weighed 54 pounds, up 20 from when she had been confiscated. She had terrible mange from head to tail and infected ears. We were told we could pick her up at noon the next day. I was praying Annie and Buddy would be OK with a new housemate.

We met the Southeast German Shepherd Rescue lady at noon at a veterinary practice about 20 minutes from our home. My account of this meeting was the beginning of documenting Sandy's story.

My heart broke as I walked into the exam room to see Sandy lying on the floor because her nails were so long she couldn't stand on a slick floor. They had been cut as far back as possible (they were curled under when she was confiscated), and she was a nervous wreck. The skin was literally hanging off her poor neck, and there was no hair on 90% of her tired body. Her mange was horrible, her poor body exhausted from trying to survive, but she had the gentlest spirit, and her look was begging someone to help her.

Michael and I went into "OK, we're going to manage this" mode, and after six prescriptions and a shot, we brought her home. She lay on her new bed in the back of the car, occasionally whimpering. I dropped Michael off with her at the playground in our neighborhood, and she could hardly walk because she was so weak.

Another reinforcement of why I don't like people who don't like animals.

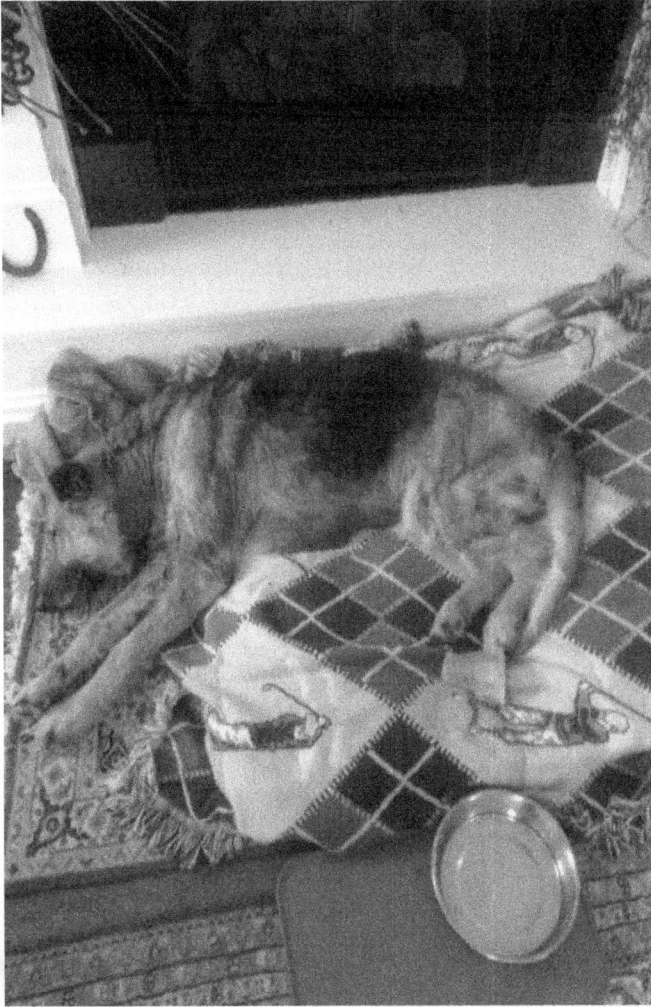

THE BEGINNING:
By Sandy

*Treat me kindly my beloved master, for no heart in all the world
is more grateful for kindness than the loving heart of mine.*

*Do not break my spirit with a stick, for though I should lick your
hand between the blows, your patience and understanding will more
quickly teach me the things you would have me to do.*

*Speak to me often, for your voice is the world's sweetest music,
as you must know by the fierce wagging of my tail when your
footstep falls upon my waiting ear.*

*When it is cold and wet, please take me inside...for I am now a
domesticated animal no longer used to bitter elements...and I ask no
greater glory than the privilege of sitting at your feet beside the
hearth...though had you no home, I would rather follow you through
the ice and snow than rest upon the softest pillow in the warmest
home in all the land...for you are my god...and I am your devoted
worshipper.*

*Keep my pan filled with fresh water for although I should not
reproach you were it dry, I cannot tell you when I suffer thirst. Feed
me clean food that I may stay well, to romp and play, and do your
bidding, to walk by your side, and stand ready, willing and able to
protect you with my life should your life be in danger.*

*And, beloved master, should the Great Master see fit to deprive
me of my health or sight, do not turn me away from you. Rather hold
me gently in your arms as skilled hands grant me the merciful boon
of eternal rest...and I will leave you knowing with the last breath I
drew, my fate was ever safest in your hands. – Beth Norman Harris*

16

January 9, 2016

It's Saturday afternoon and I'm getting ready to take a nice nap. I had the energy and strength to stand up and eat my breakfast today. And the most wonderful thing was that I went to the bathroom, down two steps to the yard all by myself. I've been inside a shelter and indoors for so long in a small concrete cage that I had to stand in the yard and look around with my eyes squinted to just breathe and check out the next-door neighbor's dog through the fence. My nice doctor gave me some Rimadyl because my ears and skin hurt so badly, and my new foster mom knew my whining was because I really hurt all over. So, she called the doctor, and she went and got me some Rimadyl. I had a great breakfast and a nice lunch. I haven't been off of my bed except to be carried into the yard until today. My foster dad was sitting on the sofa, and I went over to see if he would rub my head. He did and he didn't hit me or fuss at me so I think he likes me. My foster mom put down some funny thing on the hardwood floor that is spongy, so I went through the door they go through every night to see what is in there. I saw two other "your beds" in that room and I think that's where Annie and Buddy sleep. My foster mom cleaned my ears out again and she was really trying to be gentle. The icky stuff in my ears must be better because she didn't work on them as long as she did yesterday. I'm really sleepy now. Thank you to all my people who are sending their love my way. I never knew anybody would care about me this way. I hope it doesn't stop.

Hi, I'm Diana, Sandy's foster mom. She stood up to eat this morning and ate two cups of food. She was able to walk out of the door to the stoop and down two steps to go to the potty not once but three times today with just some encouragement but not being carried. I called the vet to get some pain meds for her as her ears were making her moan. We went out for four hours, and she was perfect while we were gone; there was no mess in the house, and she acknowledged us when we got home by holding her head up and looking at us. She ate two more cups late afternoon and another before bedtime. I've sprayed her skin every twelve hours, but it takes one-quarter of the bottle every time because there is so much mange-covered skin. I have let the vet know I need more. The Rimadyl seems to give her some relief. I did a light cleaning of her ears, and she let me gently wipe them out. They are so infected and pus-filled but actually look better than yesterday. She is more alert, and we did not have to use the lead on her tonight to go outside. She was more willing to fall asleep once bedtime came and is sleeping deeply while I write this. I want her to feel good and am impatient about the misery she has to go through before the meds really work and the skin is ok. She's getting food with probiotics and antioxidants, and vitamins, so her little body is going through quite an adjustment with antibiotics, antifungal and pain meds and topical ear ointment.

January 10, 2016: (Second full day with us)

She slept all night and got up on her own this morning to go outside. She manages the brick steps but it is still very hard for her to come up the steps. I am concerned that her very long nails are part of her discomfort, so I will talk to the vet on Monday. I ordered a Dremel for pets so I can work on them if she will let me. I cleaned her ears out pretty thoroughly. Her right ear is the most sensitive, and she moans if it gets uncomfortable while I clean it. It is definitely looking better with less pus and more just plain brown infection and sloughing off of bad skin. Her left ear is still a bit pus-filled but she let me clean it out and put drops in both. She was able to give her head a full shake without falling over. Her skin still itches and she tries to scratch behind her ears with her hind paws but just isn't strong enough to manage it. She ate a total of 5 cups of food today and her digestive system is working better. She is getting fed three to four times a day, and she eats gently and willingly. We are crushing up the meds and putting them into her food. She is holding her head up more, and she looks at us with more recognition. She does better going outside with Michael. Her tummy seems full but the hanging skin will take a while to fill out. The mange is caused by an autoimmune problem so she is getting probiotics in her food. Tomorrow, we are installing a shower head that has an attached hose so we can bathe her in our walk-in shower. She has to have at least two baths a week. She fell asleep all stretched out and seems to know she is safe.

My best day in a very, very long time. I didn't feel like I needed to wrap myself up into a ball to be safe because I think these people like me. I have gotten really good food for three days in a row and I can't remember the last time that happened. My nails are so long that it hurts me to walk so my foster mom is going to talk to my doctor about them. I actually was able shake my head today without falling over when I got medicine in my ears. My skin still itches terribly but I get a medicated bath again tomorrow. I don't know where they will put me in the bath. I'm getting a lot of medicine but it's mixed up in my food and so far it isn't bothering me. My ears feel a little better. I'm not strong enough to scratch them with my hind leg yet but I sure would like to. But the good news is that I'm not all balled up outside in the rain and I've decided it's time to stretch out and say good night. To all the people who have liked my page and who are praying for me to get better, please don't stop because I think it's beginning to work a little.

January 10, 2016

Today I had a visit from the wonderful lady who came to the shelter to keep them from putting me down. I walked around the yard for her and she was so happy and it made her cry. I had more energy this morning than I do tonight. It was not a fun afternoon because I had to have a bath for my skin treatment. I don't know why my fosters think going in that big glass box and standing under water is any fun. But my foster mom had put down mats so I wouldn't slip and a lot of dirt -or whatever it was- came off. It made me really tired and stressed me out but I still ate and even wagged my tail when patted. My rescue lady and my foster mom took a funny-looking long thing that buzzed and held it against my toenails today. It didn't hurt but they say we will have to do this every few days to get my toenails short enough that I can walk right. I guess I am staying here for a while because I also got a clean "your bed". I feel bad for the little buddies that were still at the shelter and wonder if they got a rescue too. My rescuer, Southeast German Shepherd Rescue, truly snatched me up at my last hours. They've spent over $1,500.00 on me. I never knew I was even worth a dime. They get their funds through donors; that's how they found my foster mom and dad. So, if you ever wonder if that thing they call donations really works, I'm still alive and I can't believe I am not put out in the cold like I used to be. I can't believe that I get lots of good food, I can't believe I get patted instead of pushed away. My foster parents wonder if the sadness in my eyes will ever go away. I wish I could tell them I'm just scared to hope. Thank you Facebook friends for loving me and for every thought you send my way. I think with your prayers and more days like the last three I just might be able to hope again.

We weren't sure at all she would make it through the weekend but her eyes are determined, and beneath the mange and the broken spirit, we are beginning to see a hint of hope in her eyes and her soul. It has given us the realization that this healing will be a full-time effort and that to give her any quality of life, she will need so much medical attention. But, by looking at her eyes, we can tell she has the will to live. And so, we will soldier forward with her in this battle to restore her to a life of love and quality. My emotions are so full of complete disdain for the person who chained and neglected her. Her life has to be more meaningful now. Maybe her Facebook page will increase awareness, and even if one person adopts or fosters an animal or volunteers at a shelter because of her page, it is worth it to document this journey.

January 11, 2016

I'm on my way to a long night's rest after two major accomplishments today! I saw my FD (here on known as my foster dad) eating lunch while sitting on the couch. It smelled really good so I got up and went over to ask him for some. It didn't work, but I tried. A little later I was minding my own business on my "your bed" and my FM (foster mom) started paying a lot of attention to Annie and rubbing her. I wanted in on that action so I got up and walked over to make sure my FM shared the love with me.

It was really cold outside and I'm so used to being left out that I like looking at the sky and walking on the yard. But it was so cold and windy that my FM wouldn't let me stay out because I don't have any fur on my back. She gives me this brown pill every day around 4:00 and it makes me feel better. My muscles are so weak and my hind legs don't want to hold me up, but my FPs (Foster Parents) have put down long runners of shelf lining so I don't slip on the hardwood floors. My FM got one of those buzzing things in the mail today so I'm betting it has something to do with my toenails.

I know I don't smell very good because of skin problems and the ear infections but my FPs love me anyway. I love my "your bed" and love all of you for sending me your care and kind thoughts and prayers.

We have never seen toenails this long on a dog. It must be so painful to walk and to try to pull herself up. Our hardwood floors are unmanageable for her. I resorted to pieces of shelf liners to place between the rugs from room to room. After realizing I could use yoga mats, I got them ordered. Her ear infections are requiring cleaning twice a day, but I think the antibiotics are beginning to work. Thank goodness I have small fingers and she lets me clean them with cotton pads even though I know it must hurt her.

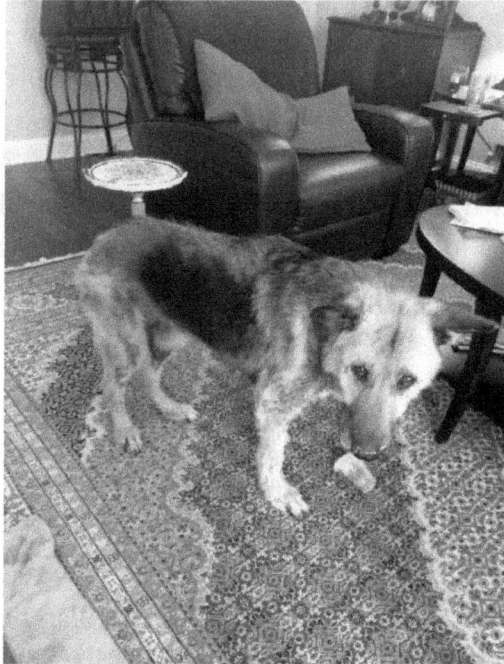

January 12, 2016

Today I've been a really good girl! I got up on my feet to eat all of my meals and I can't believe my tummy is not aching and empty anymore. My FPs are so nice to me and I have gone to the sofa several times to get head rubs. It is really cold out and I don't stay out long when I go but my FM says we have to walk around tomorrow for two minutes so I can try to build up some strength in my hind legs. Guess what! Some hair is growing back on my paws and my chin so I look like I have the beginnings of a goatee. And my FM used that buzzy thing to get a little off of my nails again. My skin stays sort of sticky because of the spray my FPs use on my skin, and it doesn't help me smell any better. My FM told my FP that I have to go in that big glass box again to have water sprayed on me. Last time it completely wore me out; I stress over new things and even new rooms to go in. There are rooms in the house I probably won't see for a while yet because I have to be able to walk well to get there. And today my FM got just a little brown stuff out of my ears and no more pus.

I can't believe there are thousands of you who have liked my page and I am so thankful for every one of your blessings and prayers. Since I'm 10 years old, I think maybe this year 2016 might be the best I've ever had. I can't thank you enough for every donation to me and every prayer and thought you send my way. But I can send you this picture to show you that you have helped me get better.

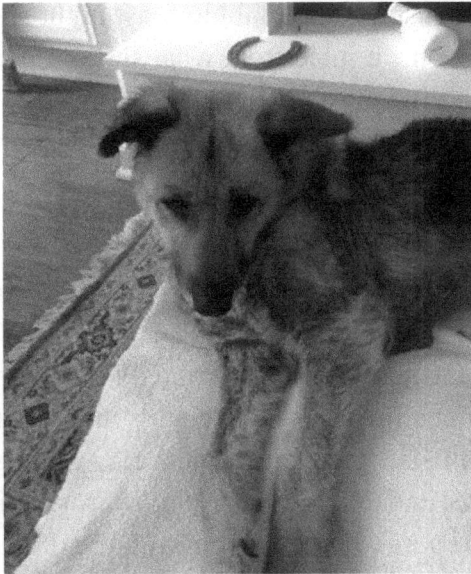

So many people are reading her story on Facebook. And because of so many requests to do so, I set up a GoFundMe site for Sandy. The outpouring of love and wanting to help is astounding and humbling. Although I had second thoughts about doing a page for her, I know now that a Power greater than me has a hand in this rescue. The

messages of love and healing are incredible. How can there be so many who love her without ever seeing or meeting her? There must be a purpose for this. I feel a great responsibility to her and to the rescue of animals. The support expressed to her and us is overwhelming.

January 13, 2016

When I got up with my FP this morning I went outside and then came in and was wondering where my FM was. It worries me, but I went into where they sleep and she was there! I was so relieved. I even went back to check again after a few minutes. I think I'm tired of this yucky wet food. My FM mixes kibble in the blender to make it soft. She thinks I don't know my pills are in there! Ha! I figured that out so now I think I'd rather just have the kibble. Last night she gave me my pill in some delicious meat juice from what she says was meat loaf. Now that's the way to give me a pill! I've got a busy day ahead. Thank you for your thoughts and prayers and for your donations on my behalf.

On to the big glass box thing........

Banner day!!!!! My FD put me on a leash to walk me around the yard to build up muscle in my hind legs. I LOVE BEING ON A LEASH and got to show him how trained I am to go with him!!! And, I wasn't hungry at all when I woke up this morning and waited quite a while to eat, but I also knew those white pills were ground up in there! Ha ha! Now I am one tired girl and got my brown pill because my FM thinks I might be sore tomorrow from walking. I did show my FM that I like to pull things out of trash cans. See, they now realize that's how I must have gotten some food and found morsels when my ribs started to show and I got so thin. My FPs made a follow-up appointment at my vet on Monday so I will also get to see my rescuer. That makes me happy. I'll be so glad when I can just be a dog strong enough to walk around and sniff and ask for head rubs without being so unsteady on my feet. My skin is still bare, but my legs have begun to heal a little. My skin was so bare and my hind end so skinny that I could not sit down because it hurt so much. I sat on my "your bed" today for the first time! Not long, but I sat. My FPs say it will be a while before I have a coat of fur on my back, but I'm getting probiotics and vitamins and tomorrow I get coconut oil rub down on my skin. I just want to know this isn't going to end. I feel like maybe I can hope.

All of you people who are sending me your prayers and love...... I can't comprehend so much love. My FM worries about me all the time and keeps telling me she wants my eyes to sparkle. Thank all of you for every single thought and every single prayer. My rescue organization will continue to pay for my meds until I am adopted, and there will come a point I hope that someone wants me for good, and will adopt me. I'd be dead without all of you. One day, when the sun is shining, and the weather is warm I want to go out in my yard and bark at the trucks and strangers and stare at the moon and send love to all of you.

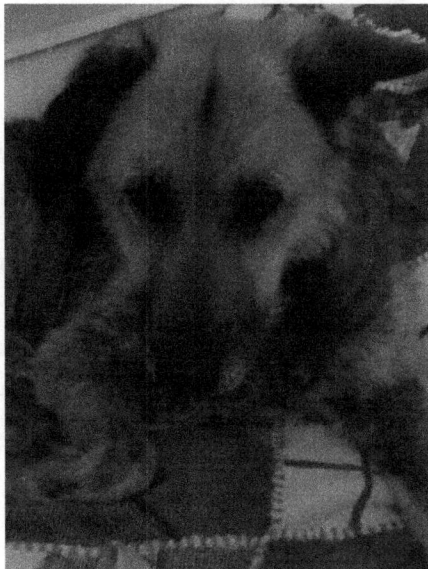

I've been thinking all day that I just must get Sandy healthy and happy. She deserves to live out her life in such love. I cannot believe how loving and tolerant she is of our other two dogs, Annie and Buddy, and of our cats, Tipper and Lulu. There is not an aggressive bone in her body. This, of course, makes me even madder at the pond scum that kept her in such horrible conditions. This girl is determined and has even begun to show a stubborn streak. That means to me she is willing to fight to be well. My observation of her, after having dogs and picking up strays for more years than I care to count, is that she is such a German Shepherd! She follows my every movement with her eyes. Nothing gets by her. She learns quickly and becomes more aware every day. And she is slowly claiming me as her own. I know there will come a time when the rescue organization will want me to turn her over…… but I'll think about that later.

January 14, 2016

It's been a busy day. I'm all clean, I have a clean bed and my tummy is full. My FM is almost asleep and I just want to tell you all how much I appreciate every single word of encouragement and every whisper of my name; I think it's the first time I've let myself be happy.

I'm going to wake up tomorrow and try hard not to be afraid and hope!

I figured out a way to keep her safe in the shower without holding her up between my legs. I take two cotton bath mats and put them on the floor of the shower with the drain in between them. I put shelf liner underneath them, so they don't slip. Now she can go in and sit while I use the handheld sprayer to bathe her. What a help this is!

January 15, 2016

I'm just really worn out tonight but it's because I walked farther early this afternoon than I have in a long time. I walked a whole block with my foster brother and sister. I keep amazing my FPs with my leash manners. I got my second rubdown of coconut oil today and I've decided I really like it! It makes my itchy skin calm down and I don't bite at my legs and sides so much. My FM found a strange lump on my hind leg so we will see the vet on Monday. It doesn't bother me, but I think it must bother her. My FD is the best and takes me outside to make sure I don't fall down every time I go to the door. He's always there to help me and I like walking on a leash with him because he has such a gentle touch and knows not to pull on me and to just ask me to do something. He's a pretty quick learner.

My days are pretty routine now except for walking more. I felt pretty good this morning and wish my skinny body had more energy and strength to hold me up. I'm beginning to think I won't ever be able to hold my right ear up again because of all the scar tissue from scratching it with my hind leg and or from frostbite. I used to be able to balance and do that, but my FPs tell me I'm beautiful and I'm even getting hugs around the neck and kisses on top of my head!!!!!! My FD had to confess to my FM that while she was out late afternoon, he gave me my food in his hand. See, I wasn't very interested in eating and he was trying to get me to eat so when he put the food in the palm of his hand and held it out to me, I felt like I'd hurt his feelings if I didn't eat it. The first bites did taste pretty good so I just went ahead and let him feed me. My FM told him it wasn't a good thing to do because I need to eat out of my bowl ....but I'm wondering if that is true because she fed me with a big spoon the first three days.

At night I am so tired and I ache so I'm hoping the vet will let me have some more brown pills. I get so weak at night and my legs just don't want to hold me up. So, I'm on a steady diet with no increase

27

because my legs have to be strong enough to hold my body and my FPs say it's going to take a while. I'm impatient to be healthy. But I've decided I want to live, I want to walk, I want to be one of the family and I want to share my inner strength and soulfulness. I may be old but I'm just starting to live.

These days my biggest wish is to keep waking up on my "your bed" and to see my FPs when I wake up. I have a little raincoat now, thanks to one of you, so my back doesn't get soaked on a night like this. Thank you for helping me with your thoughts and prayers and for your support of my rescue.

Until tomorrow. My eternal gratitude!

Meant to add this to my post for today. Look at my legs! I'm getting fur!

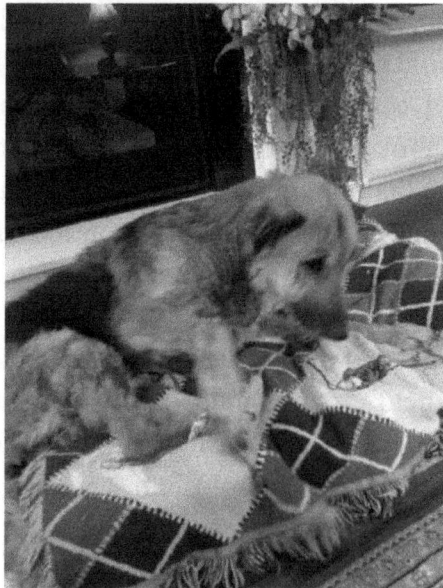

We are into a fairly established routine now. Sandy has become accustomed to her bed, and her internal clock knows exactly when it's time to eat. Our kitchen counter has become partly a pharmacy with

all her meds, lotions, cleaners and salves. She loves lying in front of the fireplace. She's the sweetest, most appreciative soul.

January 16, 2016

I loved the beautiful weather today! I hated that stupid raincoat I had to wear last night! My FM added a new food to my diet.....she thinks it has all the same ingredients as the other food but I don't think so and tried my best to be a little finicky, but she caught on. I did the three stairs to the other part of the yard today and got to smell a lot of new places and walk around for a while. Annie and Buddy seem to like to woof at people that walk by the fence, but that seems rather silly to me so I didn't. My FD is my outside buddy and my FM is my nails, skin, and ears and bath buddy. I got a total body rub today with coconut oil so I look like a canine version of John Travolta in Grease! Speaking of nails...mine were about 3" long when I was rescued so getting them down gradually is a process because it would make my nails bleed if they got too much off at a time. So, the buzzy thing came out again today and my FM says we've only got another time or two and they'll be short enough for them not to hurt me when I walk on hard floors.

And another thing.....my FPs moved my water and food bowls further from my bed because now they know I can get up to get it and they say I have to build up something called muscles in my back legs. Apparently, I don't have any "muscle tone", whatever that means. I have now learned to eat out of a bowl, and my FPs think I must have just eaten off of the ground for a long time because it took me some time to get used to the bowl. I think they are right but I'm trying to forget those awful days. My skin is getting better, and it's making my "your bed" really dirty so my FM has to wash my blanket every day. It stays over my "your bed" all the time except when she takes it away to be washed.

My FM wants to make sure I tell all of my loving friends on Facebook that she appreciates all of you too! I'm so much better in just a week, and my dreams are much better than the sleepless nights I spent feeling like I wanted to die rather than be in the cold and rain. I'm not strong enough yet to scratch myself again, and my FPs say it's a good thing because my ears need time to heal. And yes, when those cotton things come out and that white bottle comes towards me I summon the strength to get up and try to go to the backdoor.....but it never works because SHE catches up with me and cleans out my ears twice a day. She says the good news is that it looks like we can start doing it once a day. Whew!

Love is a strange thing. I can't believe how much better it has made me feel and how nice it is to know I'm warm and comfortable because of love. My tummy is full, I have all the water I want, and I even get these things called "treats". All of this because of love. If I could give each of you a big lick I would. I love all of you. I hope my loving you will make you better like you loving me has made me better.

She's so smart. She's figured out the ear-cleaning bottle and recognizes it's time to clean ears. She's even trying to get away from it. She's not really fond of the Dremel. She hates the noise and has started trying to hide her paws when that comes around. Some of her personality is beginning to show. I'm sure she will get used to the raincoat, and it is a wonderful coat at that. It was sent by one of her loving Facebook followers and is just a top-of-the-line addition to help keep her dry.

January 17, 2016

I'm going to post this early tonight, or earlier, because I have a big day tomorrow. I have to go back to my vet for a check-up and to make sure I don't have anything my FM calls "worms". So, I have to have a bath to get all the dead skin off and the coconut oil off so I don't look like a jar of Vaseline. My FD is faithful about going outside with me and took me for a short walk today. It was really cold and my coat doesn't cover my whole back so I was ready to get back inside.

New discovery today. I don't like fish, Sandy I am. I do not like it in a dish. I do not like it in a hand. I do not like it, Sandy I am. I do not like it if it's wet, I do not like it with an egg. I will not like it if you beg. I will not like it with a yam, I do not like it, Sandy I am!

So, my FM gave up and went back to my probiotic chicken...... I won!

My right hind leg doesn't want to work sometimes and gives out under me if I don't watch out. I got in a hurry today to go back to my "your bed" after adventuring into the kitchen on the yoga mats. There were too many people in there, Annie and Buddy and my FD, because there was bacon in the oven. Well, my right hind leg didn't want to come with me so I struggled a little to get where I could have a soft landing. Then later my FD took me for a walk and my leg started working better.

One of the kitties has started sitting near me. She's very calm and must think she's a dog because she doesn't react to me at all. No fun! The other kitty is just nuts. She runs through the room and up and down the hallway like her tail is on fire. She tries to climb the walls, and chases her tail like she's about to find something. I just ignore her. I think she might have a screw loose.

My FM says Annie and Buddy are going with me in the car so I don't get stressed tomorrow. Hope they sit in the very back so I can lie on my "your bed".

My joints ache tonight and I'm slow getting up. Maybe my FPs will serve me dinner in bed (yay).

Your love and prayers are important now because this is not a sprint but a marathon. Thankful I have my FPs and all of you! Many of you have sent my rescue things for me. I cannot ever repay you but hope you know how much it means to me.

The outpouring of love and support for Sandy on her page and in cards and items to help her is astounding. I am feeling so blessed to be part of this miracle.

January 18, 2016

This day has been...different. It started early with a walk around the yard, then a bath, then a ride to see my vet. He was pleased about the progress I've made and I have gained weight and weighed in at 73.8 pounds. I've got some more new pills for my skin and my ears are looking so much better. Still work to do and I've discovered that I like the salmon and sweet potato no grain food! Yay, no more of that other kind of fish!

One of my angels named Kristine sent me a new blanket to lie on along with probiotic treats and a puppet nutter bone!! My rescuer brought them to me when she met my FPs at the vet! I'm so happy and I'm already curled up in my new blanket in front of the fire in the fireplace. How did she know I needed these? Thank you, my angel, and all the other angels I have out there who love me and send me healing energy.

I have to tell you I was terrified when my FD put me in the car today. I had visions of going back to the shelter and being alone and cold and hungry. I whimpered but realized that Annie and Buddy got in the car too so it gave me a little comfort. I was so glad to see my rescuer, and I was so relieved when my FD PUT ME BACK IN THE CAR!!!!!! I came back to my "your bed" and a fancy new cuddly blanket.

And, my FM has started giving me my pills in this really good stuff so I don't even taste the medicine. I am so lucky to have a rescuer and can't but think about all of my brothers and sisters who don't have a foster parent and need one so badly. I am a work in process, and I will never be perfect, but my FM says nobody is perfect so I'll be ok with that. Even my FP's neighbor wants me to walk to see her when I get better. Who knew so many people would care about me? My FM says this whole deal is a joy for her. I'm not sure what that means but I guess she thinks the money they spend on me is worth it. That's amazing!

I'm ready for a nice warm sleep. I love you all!

January 19, 2016

I'm a dog!!!!! I got to do real dog things today!!! Even though it is bitter cold, I went out with a wonderful coat on (that one of you sent me) with Annie and Buddy. It really looked silly because I'm longer than it is but it sure kept me warmer than I would have been without it!!! I got to sniff and walk around and even smelled the dog next door through the fence! Who knew I'd ever live to see a day when I went out multiple times on my own, and met my FM at the door when she came in tonight! It was all pretty exciting and I really like my new food. So yes, if salmon is a fish, I like it, but if it tastes like a fish or smells like a fish, I don't. My tail doesn't work yet, and my FPs are hoping that as I gain muscle tone in my hind quarters that it will work again. It just sort of hangs there right now. I've worn myself out with getting up and down so I am headed to my "your bed" for a nice warm sleep. I can't believe I'm not outside in the cold; that's where I was for a long time and it's no wonder I have such bad skin. But, my nails are much better because of that buzzy thing. And when my FM comes with that thing again, I'm going to get up and walk away!

Your kind prayers and loving thoughts are helping me get so much better. Please say a prayer for all my brothers and sisters who are out in the cold and who will die in the winter storm that is coming. If you have any doubt about fostering and the help it can be just use my name as a reference. Rescue the perishing, care for the dying. Even one day of love might save one of our lives.

Love to all of you and my heart is so grateful!

It's very cold and predicted to be frigid. Sandy has made me think of all the homeless and neglected animals that will be out in it. There is so much to do to save them. My involvement with Best Friends as a volunteer opened my eyes several years ago. Maybe Sandy can help more people be aware of how rewarding it is to save a dog. I am amazed at the number of friends she now has on Facebook. It gives me renewed faith in humanity every day.

January 20, 2016

I'm all warm and cozy and ready for the winter storm. I've been really tired today but still able to go out and do the steps on my own. There's a new dog next door and he and Buddy get all woof-woof at the fences. I don't know why.... he's no big deal to me. I just laugh at their thinking they are all that! My FPs won't let me stay out very long because I'm pretty hairless down my back. I got my coconut oil treatment today. I like to lick it so my FM says the next time I'm only getting it where I can't lick (we will see about that).

Keep praying that all my animal friends are safe and warm. Your caring and sharing really makes a difference to me and to all the abused, abandoned and neglected fur babies out there.

My FD is preparing for the winter stuff and says for me not to worry, that he will make sure the steps aren't slickery.

Before I nod off again, I just have to tell all of you that my story has reached all the way to Scotland and Australia!! I have people loving me from the United Kingdom, Canada, and about every state in the USA. You see, each of you does make a difference! I even got someone to commit to being a foster parent. Without a rescue like mine so many of us would be killed or die in the cold and damp. Your love and your prayers send healing to me every day. The positive energy that I receive through your love is solid evidence that you make a difference. You see, without all of you I would have no voice, I would have no choice.

"Bless the Beasts and the Children". We are all the essence of God. I am in the light of a new life because you love me. You have more love to share and I hope my brothers and sisters will always find a place in your hearts like I did.

Sleep peacefully. I will.

Sandy

It's so amazing. The sharing and caring that have been the result of Sandy sharing her story on Facebook. It's hard to believe so many people have responded. It makes my heart glad and hopeful. Sometimes, when I'm so tired of bathing her and cleaning her up, I think about the privilege I've been granted to care for this sweet soul. I don't ever want to lose sight of that.

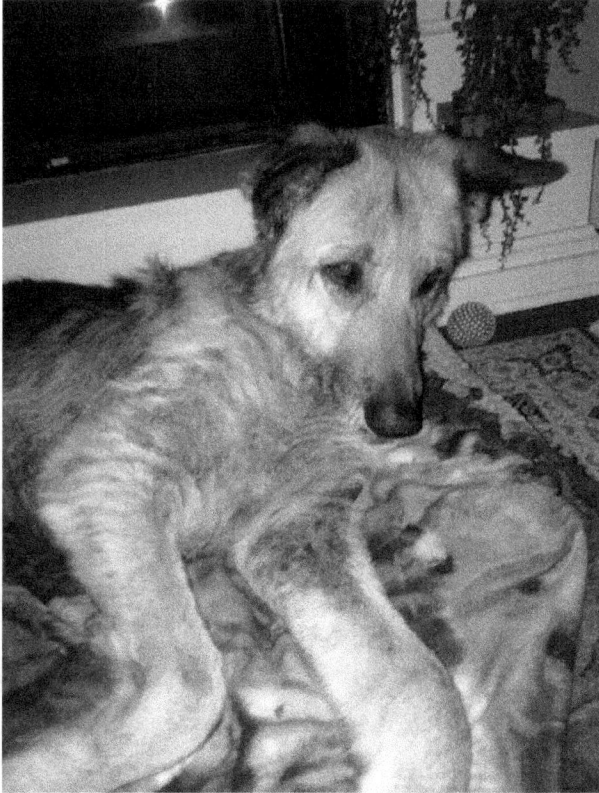

January 21, 2016

My sweet loving friends from all over the world: I am so humbled and so blessed to have your support and your love. I never knew this much love was possible, never ever even hoped it would come to me. My FM says she can't believe my story has touched the hearts of so many and healed her heart in many ways. I just have to list some of the places where my loving extended family lives: Denmark, Sweden, Singapore, New Zealand, Australia, Scotland, the United Kingdom, Spain, South America, Michigan, Oregon, Vermont, California, and almost every state in the USA.

On my health.... I walked today with my FD on a longer walk than ever. I loved the smell of the crisp air and the frozen ground. I love walking with him because he never yanks on me or yells at me. I take my dear sweet time and no one ever hurries me. My FPs are really concerned about my back legs because they go skittering out from underneath me easily and my hind end goes crooked when I first try to walk. My tail is not working and I do not like it being touched. It's sore right where it connects to my body and my FPs think I must have an injury to my back end. I moan when lie down because it is uncomfortable to get situated. Once I get there though I'm ok. I managed to get up and greet my FPs when they got home from the store. Seems my FD is very concerned about me getting out during the winter storm, so he got some special stuff to put on the walkway that is pet safe. Annie has learned to leave my food bowl alone even if it has stuff in it, but Buddy will snatch it in a nano second. He got the loud voice today when he got caught. I'm a nibbler so the other two have to know to leave my food alone! I don't get upset because I now know there's more where that came from....but my FM says that Annie will be a fat girl and Buddy will be a piggy boy if they keep it up!

Bath day tomorrow....... Glass box here I come.

Big news! I have tiny little hairlettes on my back. Off to my "your bed" and my nice warm soft dreams.

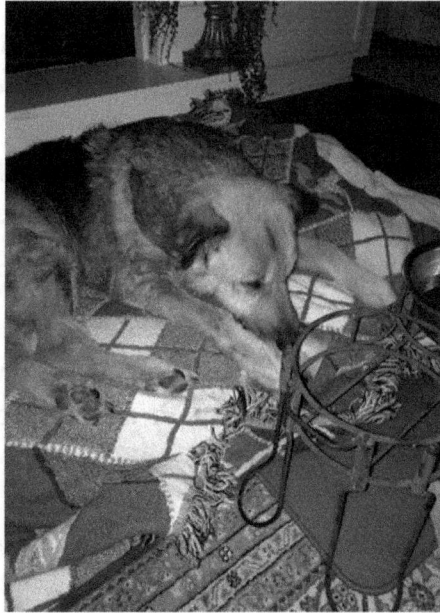

January 23, 2016

First icy snowy day I ever remember when I was warm inside by the fireplace! I've had to go outside several times today and it's really awful. My FD put down some stuff on the steps and walkway that is pet safe and melts the ice .... Sort of. I'm not fond of this weather.

But, I was such a good girl today! It was bath day and I got in the big glass box all by myself and had the best bath ever with warm soapy stuff and my FM's gentle rubbing and rinsing. My skin is turning from black to pink in spots all over my tummy, but my neck is still black from the mange I have. The good news is that I don't itch anymore and my FM says it will be a few months before my neck looks better.

I also got a chance to show my FPs that I like a tennis ball. I'm not strong enough to jump up and get it or to catch it but I love holding it in my mouth and squeezing it. I put some pictures of me with my ball on Facebook.

Ok...it's hard enough for me to walk on normal ground, but on all this snow and ice is ridiculous. You won't believe what my FD did for me! He took a pickaxe and chopped all the ice off of the steps to both sides of the yard and shoveled pathways for me to use. I've been able to go out and walk around and watch the little birds and stick my nose through the fence. My FD even took me for a slickery walk but we went very slowly. My FM double blanketed me (she learned that from her daughter and the horses!) and I was warm as toast except for my feet and tail. The big news today is that my FM got me to play tug of war.... I gave her two big tugs but had to quit because my hind legs were all wobbly.

Yes, I still have no fur on my neck and chest and belly but with the superfood and the supplements I'm getting I think it will be only a few months. I get glucosamine and MSM and my FM added flax seed to meds today. I will be so glad when I can sit down. My tail or hind quarters are too sore or skinny still.

You know, my story is a pretty good one, at least the rescue part is. But there are thousands of us with stories just waiting for rescue. Many rescues are already rehabilitated and don't need anything but a loving home and warm bed. My FM says she had thought about fostering before but always thought it would be too much. Then, when I was on death row, sitting in a cage in a concrete floor, not able to even stand, a lady named Sandra made a connection with me. She called Southeast German Shepherd Rescue and they said they would try to find a foster but they had 2 days to do it before I was killed. SGSR called my FM and she couldn't say no. I'm so lucky. And I'm not a healthy girl and need a lot of time to heal but she said yes.....and here I am. My nails were almost 3" long, I had mange over 85% of my body, I ached, I itched, my ears were filled with infection, and I really had given up. I smelled just plain awful. Now, even though I can't stand up long, and my skin is still bare, my ears feel great, I love being able to eat, I have fresh water and no one ever hits me or yells at me. I have heat and comforts I never had before. And I have all of you pulling for me. There really are some good people in this world. Sometimes you have to be in the deepest darkest places before the sunshine comes. My biggest wish is for people like my FPs to SAVE THEM ALL, and help with the national campaign being organized by Best Friends to have no homeless pets by 2022. Please visit www.bestfriends.org to join this effort.

January 24, 2016

Nope, no new fur except on my legs. Some tiny hairlettes on my back but nothing but bare skin on my neck and chest and tummy. The mange didn't get to my shoulder, but I'd begun to lose the black hair on my saddle markings. It looks and feels better and isn't coming out now that I'm getting lots of nourishment. My skin and hair problems are all because my auto-immune system had shut down so badly. I'm getting some stuff for my joints and hips that my FM gives the other pups in the house and I get flax seed and coconut oil in my food and probiotic treats, and now she hopes to start giving me some really good antioxidants. I get an egg once a day too. It's just going to take several months to grow hair. I'm going for X-rays on my tail soon. No, I didn't run today. That would be nothing short of a miracle. But I did go for a walk, and those make me tired, but I do better every day. The picture that looks like I'm panting was taken when my FM was playing with me and a toy so I had my mouth open.

My rescue organization has been wonderful about making sure I have what I need. So many of you have sent me love and presents and

I feel pretty special. There are a lot of my brothers and sisters on rescue sites all over the country. Please save, don't buy. They all need forever homes and you can shop on Amazon Smile and pick your rescue to support through your purchases.

I found the living room today! On my own!! I was following one of the kitties (I find they are very curious creatures) and lo and behold, there it was..... another room! My FPs are watching something on the wall and my FP keeps talking to it like he thinks someone is stupid. Glad it's not me! The thing on the wall talks and makes a lot of other sounds.....but whatever is going on, my FD thinks they can hear him. I don't think so because they never answer. Full tummy, warm fire, comfy!

January 25, 2016

Walking, resting, eating, walking, sleeping, eating. My legs are a bit stronger and today I got to walk with Annie and Buddy. Buddy is very well-mannered on leash. Annie is hard-headed and pulls so my FM was walking them and me with my FD. It's time for the buzzy thing and I think my FM will try it again tomorrow. See, I've gotten strong enough to pull away and get up and GET AWAY.

My legs are getting fluffier and my FM thinks I need protein and skin supplements. Getting coconut oil in my food now, so I am not getting it on my skin. Itching isn't too bad and I think I smell better.

I do have a favorite toy, and one day I'm going to be strong enough to shake it really hard! Right now, I just make sure I put it near my "your bed" and sometimes I toss it in the air without even standing up. I think maybe some of my brothers and sisters who were with me in the dark place have gone over the Rainbow Bridge; don't know for sure but have a feeling.

All of you are so kind to me, and I can't believe people can be so nice. The mean person who had me before just didn't care that I was starving and suffering. He didn't care that I didn't have water or that I couldn't walk. He didn't care that I ached or that I felt such despair, or that being chained on cold cement made me want to die. Now I have all the love and prayers anybody could ever want or need. It's so unbelievable. I've slept warm and been fed for almost 3 weeks. Three weeks out of nine or ten years. I wonder why that person ever wanted me in the first place. I only hope all the puppies I had are in warm loving homes.

She has made such progress. From being unable to stand to now showing some spirit and a desire to trust us. Late at night, I sit and weep about the awful life she had, and how inhuman her treatment was. I hope that I never understand that kind of treatment of an animal, because hating that treatment is my passion.

Please, please pray for my foster cousin Bozzie. He lost use of his back legs this afternoon and is at emergency vet for MRI in the morning. His sister just went over the Rainbow Bridge on this past Thanksgiving Day. Her name was Maggie. So, I figure if all your prayers and love can help me, I'd ask you to send love and prayers to Bozzie tonight. My FA (foster aunt) and FU (Foster Uncle) are very worried. Please send prayers their way too. Thank you to all those who love me!

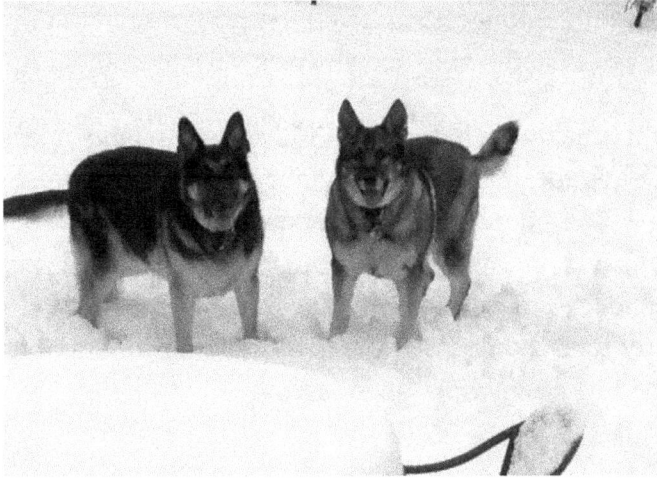

Boz on left. Maggie on right.

January 26, 2016

Please keep prayers coming for my foster cuz Bozzie. They are working and I am so grateful. Bozzie says for me to tell you how grateful he is! My FM says never doubt the positive energy and healing that comes with prayer! Just look at me!!!!

Love all of you,

Sandy

Later that same day

My foster cousin Boz has a herniated disc and is in surgery as I write this. The prognosis is hopeful. And all your love and healing energy has helped, I just know it!!! My FA and FU will have 6 to 8 weeks of helping him recover but he is a well-loved dog and has been his whole life! He still needs your prayers as so many of us do.

I went on the longest walk yet, today! I'm tired but my spirits are good! I even licked Annie and she was very nice about it.

Isn't it amazing what love and healing thoughts and prayers do? My FM says the positive energy speaks to the universe and things beyond her understanding happen in the way of blessings, coincidence, or default...... I'm not sure what that all means but she says she hopes I'm an example. Speaking of example... I got another egg on my food today. I'm more active asking for attention and today I gave me FM doggy licks and kisses!

January 26, 2016

How do I thank you for all you mean to me and for all the wishes and love you have not only sent to me but also to my fosters and even my foster cousin? This huge outpouring of love and healing energy is truly miraculous. Those who love me have no idea what I have come through in 3 weeks and it is because of their prayers and support. You know what I was thinking today? That if I reached over 40,000 views this week, that if every single person who viewed my page would send $1.00 to a rescue they could rescue and foster and pay for medical bills for almost 20,000 dogs. Isn't that incredible...... My story and my loyal supporters could save 20,000 or more like me who were one step away from the needle of silence. Isn't that unbelievable? Can you imagine being part of saving the lives of that many dogs? I think I'd be so happy I'd be dancing!

I did one of my favorite things I get to do just now. I'm stretched out in front of the fireplace on my "your bed" and I stretched really long and heaved a huge sigh. I hope you hug your fur babies tonight! I'm gonna hug my FPs! Thank you for all the advice about my skin. And coat. One day I'm going to be gloriously gorgeous. Love to all of you.

January 27, 2016

My FC Boz is recovering nicely and came through the surgery well. He'll be in hospital for 3 more days. Thank you for sharing your prayers with him. I was very worried that my FA and FU would go through another horrible heartbreak but your prayers surely helped!

To all my people who have asked how they can help me:

1) My page was initiated because I want so badly to make people aware of the horrible things that happen to us when we are abandoned, when people are negligent, when we are abused, when we are sick and homeless.

2) To my pure amazement and joy, many of you have wanted to help me and my brothers and sisters in need, so here is the information you've asked for:

Go to www.southeastgermanshepherdrescue.com

They are the rescue that saved my life and without them I would have been put down.

Now for the real update:

My FC Bozzie is doing great! They took his IV out tonight and took out his catheter. He is walking with only a little help and hopes he can go home on Saturday. He will have a ramp to go out to the yard for a while but they expect a full recovery! My thanks to Veterinary Referral and Clinical Care in Manakin-Sabot, VA for the expert neurosurgery and the care!!!!

And, I have little mini muscles growing in my hind legs! We practiced going up a small hill twice today and I did great. I wouldn't say I'm ready for a long walk yet but I'm getting there. I played a little today with the tennis ball and my FM was surprised that I can grab it in the air if she gives it a little bounce. Annie is a counter surfer and while my FP was gone, she took a bag of my skin and coat treats and ate EVERY SINGLE ONE. She's going to be as big as a barn if she doesn't stop stealing things off of the counter. My FM asked her what she'd done and she tucked her head and went into the bedroom. BUSTED! And now I'm settled onto my "your bed" knowing I'll get one more time to go out before bedtime and one more TREAT. Love Sandy.

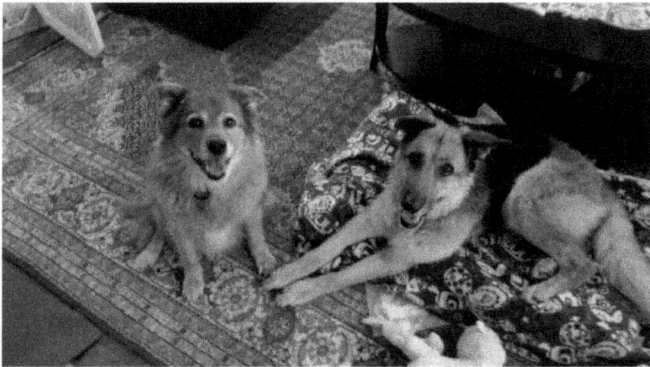

January 28, 2016

I HAVE HAIRLETTES ON MY BACK! I'm so excited because I thought I might never have my nice coat back. Do you know how many years and months and days and hours it takes to neglect someone like me to the point that they cannot walk and have mange and 3" nails and very little coat left? It was so long that I had ear infection that my FM now thinks I have some hearing damage and might have frostbite damage that makes one of my ears fold funny. Can you imagine the hours in the cold and rain, the thunderstorms and heat? And, no food and very little water. My poor body wasted away and I know we are all impatient for it to heal, but I've only had good food for three weeks and only been loved for four weeks..... out of my 9 years.

How can the humans just walk by and ignore us when we are hungry and sick? I just wonder about that a lot. Why do some people have to be just mean, only worried about themselves with no care for other creations on earth?

I don't know, and probably never will. But my FPs will wave my flag and the flag of all animals who are abused as long as they live. If you knew or even thought of one of us is being neglected or abused, what would you do?

January 29, 2016

It's Christmas at my Foster home!! I was in a shelter when December 25th happened so the special feeling I have right now must be what other pups feel when Santa comes. My wonderful Facebook family has sent me presents and my FM says I'll get a clean blanket every day now!! And I can't even begin to tell you all the wonderful things that the post elf brought to the house today! So here are other pictures and my FPs are overwhelmed by the generosity! I am so excited about the treats and toys and they are so excited about the shampoos and vitamins and nutritional stuff and even though I know what shampoo is, I'm not sure what vitamins are. But I know it all must be good for me.

What a blessing to receive so much. My FPs say we will pay it forward. I have a new fuzzy hippopotamus and I love to shake him around!

I love each of you and hope you know in your heart how grateful I am.

We celebrated Christmas in our home on the last of January. Our traditional Christmas was always held in Virginia, so gathering the immediate family had to wait until now. Sandy had no idea what all

47

the paper and shiny bows were about, but Annie and Buddy were "stocking trained" and once the stockings were stuffed and in place, they both knew Santa had left treats. Sandy caught on quickly.

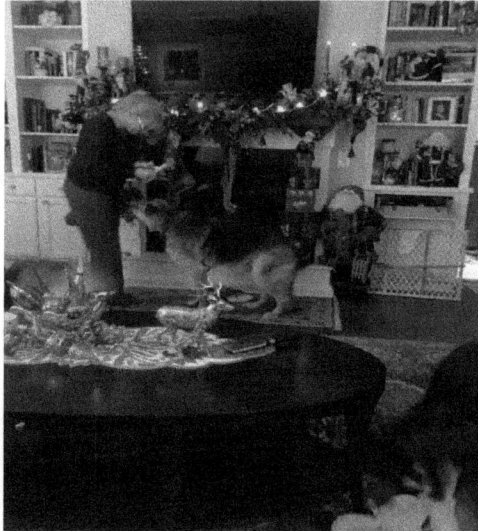

January 30, 2016

I am such a good girl that my FM gave me some of the homemade treats today three times!!!! I had a wonderful long bath complete with massage and feel a good deal better now that I have some meds for my aches. However, I must tell you that being in that glass box for a long time wears me out! After a nice nap drying in front of the warm fire, I walked around the yard a bit with the warm sun shining on me, but my FM still made me wear a coat...

Then late his afternoon I took the longest walk yet and went down to meet my new friends, Hagen and Emily. They asked if I was a police dog and my FM told them I was the same breed but that I'm just a pet. She told them the reason that I don't have hair and it made them sad. They were happy that they get to watch me get better.

My FPs say my diet is better than theirs... I sure do like eggs and my appetite today was good. My FM is so happy to have enough blankets for me that she doesn't have to wash every day!! Oh... and about that buzzy thing that they used on my nails when I was weak... well, I can get away from it now and I showed my FM how well I can do it.

Each of you who read my post is very important to me and to all the homeless, abused or abandoned, neglected and mistreated pups and kitties. If my post helps at least one of these then it makes me happy because I want to help Save Them All!

January 31, 2016

What a beautiful day it's been and I've loved being outside without a coat!! I have two doggies next door to us and loved hanging out at the fence with neighbors. My human foster sister and brother came to see me and I showed off the best I could. We are all so proud of the body mass I am gaining and my FPs are working extra hard to make sure my hind legs can carry my additional weight.

I won't be ready to be adopted until all my medical issues are clear and/or identified. My FS has her certification in canine therapy and she says my nerves appear to be good so it may be skeletal

I love getting comments from all of you and every single one gets read! I love that you spread the word of how a mangy, neglected girl like me can be restored to health with love and nurturing. I know I've heard from many of you that you've been inspired to foster or adopt or to volunteer. This news makes all of us joyful and thankful. Social media has been a true blessing for me and for others. Keep sharing and caring and together we can begin to Save Them All.

THE LEARNING

"You can't buy happiness, but you sure can rescue it."

~ Anonymous

"Does not the gratitude of the dog put to shame any man who is ungrateful to his benefactors?"

~ St. Basil

"All his life, he tried to be a good person. Many times, however, he failed. For after all, he was only human. He wasn't a dog."

~ Charles M. Schultz

February 1, 2016

I got up this morning and am pretty tired already. My FM took me for a walk to Anita's house and back. I liked meeting her and she loves us fur babies. My appetite isn't much today, and my walking wasn't as easy as yesterday so I'm going to bed early.

My FC Bozzie is getting the best care and walking slowly. He weighs 120 pounds so he's a big boy and has to be extra careful. But, thankfully, he is on the mend.

I got a nice care package today and all of you who are sending me gifts...I just can't thank you enough. I hope every good person who follows me can inspire another good person to help us all have a home.

'Til tomorrow...

February 2, 2016

Just so all my beloved friends don't worry, I am ok. I got around better today than yesterday and I ate a little better today. My FM took all three of us on a walk at the same time and it must have looked like she was doing rope tricks! Annie pulls, Buddy is slow and very leash cooperative, and I am wobbly. She says she won't do that again! Thursday is my day to go to the vet for X-rays and follow up. I'm not sure how they are going to get me in the car... so my FD will probably just pick me up.

I'm going to find that buzzy thing and chew it up so my FM can't use it anymore. She thinks if she just does one nail a day I'll learn to sit still. Not happening!

This getting better thing is slow going. I'm getting lots of vitamins and joint treats and coconut oil and eggs and probiotics. And my fur is making my back feel prickly so it must be sprouting.

Did you hear about the 600 or more animals in North Carolina who were rescued by the ASPCA FROM A HORRIBLE, HORRIBLE place? I am so glad they got rescued and hope they all get homes.

February 3, 2016

I started out the day eating well but my appetite got better and better and I have a very full tummy! And I had so much spunk I played with toys. I tried to get Annie to play but she's gotten so fat that she doesn't want to play. My FM has her on a serious diet. Every time my FM calls me I get up off of my "your bed" and walk over to her and that is really big news! My FPs are very happy about this good day. My FB (Foster Brother), Buddy, is being Mr. Aloof so my FM is letting him get on a blanket on the couch. MANIPULATION!!!

Special prayers for the people that are trying to bring an abuse case against the bad people who treated us so badly. Isn't it amazing how much positive energy and support results in good things!!

My FPs think I should run for President. They think I'd inspire people to do the right thing. But I don't think I have the right hair-do, I'm not progressive but progressing, I don't like tea, I was born in the USA, I don't speak another language, and I don't know where my children are...I don't point my paw well, and there are a lot of people I probably would sniff out in a minute!

So, I'll hang here with Mr. Aloof and Ms. Piggy.

February 5 2016

It was big glass box morning but I really did not mind because I get the best massage and it makes my skin feel so good. I don't even have that musty, mangy smell anymore and there is pink skin showing in spots on my tummy and neck.

This afternoon was really hard. I had to go to the vet to see about my tail and I hate to be picked up so I whined when I got out in the car. I got to see my Southeast German Shepherd rescuer and they were all very pleased with my coat and my skin and nails. The bad news is that I have a spinal condition from the years of neglect, and my back is very sore most all of the time. It's sort of like spinal stenosis but a cartilage problem too. I'm way too old and fragile for surgery so I will be on some new meds to relax the muscles in my back and reduce the constant pain. I was such a good girl for the vet, and the good news is that when I stop hurting I will likely be able to wag my tail. The whole trip exhausted me but my FM gave me the new meds about 20 minutes ago and I'm being monitored. I think they know I'm tired so we won't know until tomorrow if it makes me woooozie! My right ear is crinkled a bit from an old hematoma but my FPs think I'm pretty perfect just the way I am.

Years of being abused wasted away so much from my life, but I'm pretty sure the life I have left will always be filled with good things. I'm so thankful for being rescued and for people loving me. I'm so thankful for food, a "your bed", treats, coats to keep me warm and dry, a nice yard, water anytime I want it, and just being able to breathe the air and know I won't wake up on a chain. I treasure your constant blessings and all the thoughts, prayers, and energy that you create for me and all my friends who need you.

We continue to be so surprised and so thankful for all the support and kindness expressed to Sandy on her Facebook page. With all the political bickering and the news that always seems sad, we are overwhelmed by the show of love we have received. Isn't it a lesson for all of us that we can come together over the love and rescue of an animal when people in so many places are at odds?

February 5, 2016

I was so glad it wasn't a rainy soppy day, and I went out into the sunshine several times. My FPs don't know yet if the new medicine is working or making any difference but I was a bit more interested in playing and going to the door when Annie barked. I mostly rested today from the hard day yesterday.

I've decided to be sort of picky about what I eat. My FM is sometimes adding egg and coconut oil so I don't like it when she does not add it... so I don't eat it. Then she mixes it to get me to eat it and I win. It's worked pretty well but I think she's catching on.

One of the kitties in the house is so gentle and quiet and likes to hang around on the sofa. The other one is a bit off, if you ask me, and tries to eat artificial flowers and loves to hide in cabinets. She jumps up in the air and comes right back down and I can't figure out what she's doing. My FM says she's whacko. However, she's pretty amusing.

I love all the things you all say about me getting better but most of all I love it that so many of you will volunteer or rescue or foster or adopt one of us. I love it that you send my story all over the world and am so thankful for all of you sharing my story. My FPs think it is important to pay it forward so you are helping me do that each time you share my story or encourage me or think of those of us who are in harm's way and pray for us. Each one of you is a candle in the dark that becomes brighter every day...for me, and for all of us.

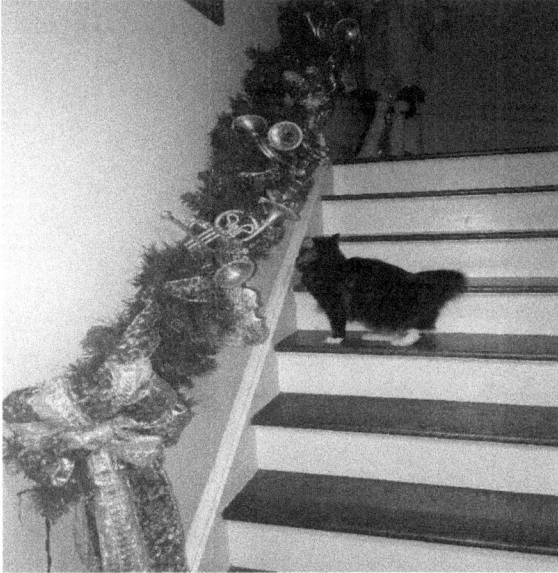

Lulu getting into mischief

February 6, 2016

Well, it happened. Sort of slow, but...I WAGGED MY TAIL! My FPs came in this afternoon from errands and I met them at the door along with Annie and Buddy...and it happened! And instead of just hanging there it is curled up a tiny bit! I think I'm definitely feeling better with the new meds! My next big move was to "trot" to the back door when I was coming in from the yard. Now, I know for some of you this doesn't seem like a big deal. But for me, I don't even remember the last time I wagged!

It's been a good day, and I know the good wishes and encouragement is helping me and it also helps my FPs! Annie and Buddy go out in the yard on their own and get around very well. But my FPs have to go with me every time I go out, and the pooper scooper is getting double duty.

Well, it's time for me to go to the debate and push for the national animal abuse registry. If you haven't signed up to petition to ask for it, just google it and join in.

THE LIVING

"If you don't own a dog, at least one, there is not necessarily anything wrong with you. But there may be something wrong with your life."

~ Roger Caras

February 7, 2016

We are watching that thing my FP talks to over the fireplace. Well, I'm not actually watching, but they are. My FM's favorite part so far was Lady Gaga singing the national anthem.

I wagged a little more today and I keep asking Buddy to play with me but he won't.

I'm really glad that the governors of Colorado and North Carolina made a bet that includes sending dog and cat food to shelters! Now they just need to work on making kill shelters illegal.

I was on a kill list and missed it by a day, only because the rescue bought me two extra days. I was so ready to die. I ached and hurt all over and I just had no hope. My back was aching, my feet so bad that I couldn't walk, my ears were full of sores, and I had no fur on my back or tummy. I was so weak I couldn't eat. My FPs fed me out of their hands for almost two weeks until I could stand to eat. My FP carried me out to the yard....

Now, I am happy. I don't ache all the time, I have regular meals, I have a coat to keep me warm, I have blankets and a "your bed" and I have kitties and Buddy and Annie. I have two FPs who love me and I have all of you. What a miracle.

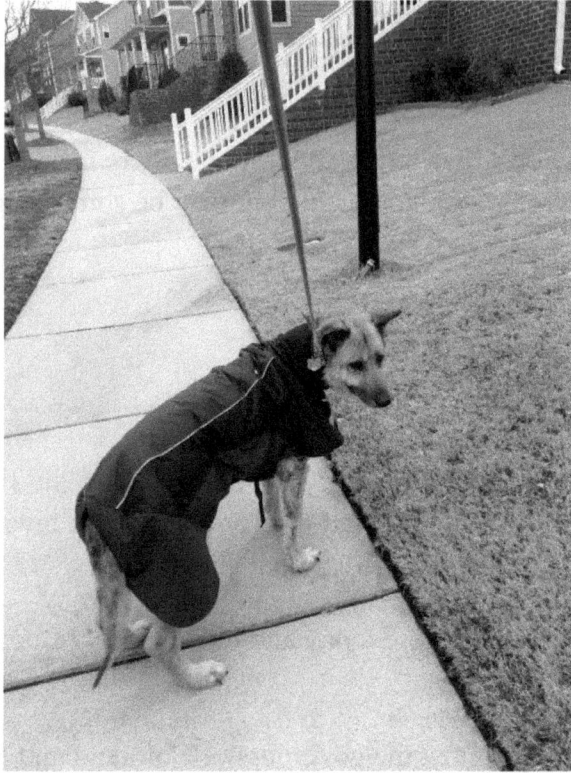

<u>February 9 2016</u>

I woke my FM up at 4:00 am because I needed to go out. You should have seen her stumbling around trying to put my coat on me. I do not think she thought it was funny. She even went back to bed so we all did. I was picky about eating breakfast but other than that it was what I've begun to think of as a normal day. I walked a long way today and worked up an appetite. Don't forget that if your dogs or kitties decide not to like the food you've bought, some shelter may need it. All the shelters always need old towels and blankets so please make an effort to drop them off.

Today my FM decided it would be a silent day of that thing over the mantle being quiet. Everyone stayed so peaceful and calm. I love sleeping in my FPs room now and am really one of the gang. Today was a coconut oil skin treatment that I love to lick off of myself if I can. Tomorrow is big glass box day and I get a nice massage that will help my FPs and my rescuer know how much I can be rehabilitated. It's really really cold out so I am very thankful for having a coat that covers me and one that my FM can just put on if I'm going out for a minute.

I can't help but think of my brothers and sisters who will freeze in this coming weather. If you see an animal left outside please call your local police or an animal rescue. My FM is working on getting a little dog in our neighborhood in from the cold. Some people are just not meant to have pets!

My walk today was good and we went up a couple of hills to help the muscles in my back legs. My mini muscleettes are growing into actual muscles. I'm still pretty thin and have a lot of loose skin on my neck and chest, my coat won't be full for another 4 to 5 months but those little hairlettes keep sprouting!

Don't forget to drop off towels and blankets at shelters!

February 10, 2016

I just got news that one of us needs special prayers and rescue. I'm just trying to pay it forward but need all of you to help me do that!

https://www.facebook.com/savinggsds/posts/461767427340396

Courtesy Post - Louisiana Shelter.

Hanani (gracious), a 6-year-old unaltered male German Shepherd. Our Animal Control department received a phone call about a stray, sick, mangy GSD that needed assistance. Our officer arrived on scene to find a most heartbreaking sight. A hunched-over, Demodex-covered, bleeding, underweight dog. She picked him up and placed him on a towel in her unit and hurried back to the shelter for our vet staff to exam. Once back at the shelter, he was given a small amount of food and given an extensive bath to help rid him of some of the buildup in his fur. The entire time he was staring with sad eyes. Hanani has been underweight at 54 lbs. He is heartworm positive on top of his other issues. He now needs a place to continue to recover. We are unable to hold him here at the shelter while he recovers due to our lack of space. I have attached pictures of him for you to view. If you can help Hanani, please contact me as soon as possible.

Shelter Supervisor/Rescue Coordinator

Terrebonne Parish Animal Shelter

131 Plant Road

Houma, LA 70360

985-873-6709 ext. 204

rbrunet@tpcg.org

www.tpcg.org/animalshelter

February 11, 2016

I am overjoyed that my poor sick friend in Louisiana has another chance thanks **to Red Stick German Shepherd** rescue in Louisiana. What a strong unity all of you have built by being so supportive of me and loving me enough to reach out and seek help for others like me…the sheer power of it is hard to comprehend and who knew that a neglected sad 10-year-old girl could bring so many loving people together. My FPs say all of you have no idea how powerful your love, your positive energy, your prayers and your voices are. Thank you for speaking up, for reaching out and for not scrolling past just another dog in need. See, every one of you makes a difference by the energy you create and that gets passed on and on and has wonder and awe packed in a powerful message.

I hope your day was good like mine. I smelled the clean, cold, fresh air. I walked, I slept, I was petted and spoken to and loved. I am warm and fed and secure. I am blessed. Who could want more, and so many yet to rescue...

February 12, 2016

Thank you, **Red Stick German Shepherd Rescue** for saving this baby. Thank you, all my friends for sharing!

So, today was a double coat day. My FM made me wear one over another because it is really pretty cold here and I'm still hairless in many places. I had a wonderful massage by a professional on Wednesday and she taught my FM how to work on my vertebrae in my tail and the muscles in my hind legs. My whole body got massaged today and it was wonderful!

I am eating a normal amount every day now and that means my body isn't in starvation mode anymore. The skin on my tummy is beginning to get pink and a lot of the black is going away. The two baths a week thing is working, and it ought to be if I have to get in that glass box all the time!

We are all prepared for any snow and ice we may get; the snow shovel is outside the door and the walkways have all that PETSAFE de-ice stuff on them.

One of the kitties, and I know which one, must be really bent out of shape with the attention I'm getting because she tinkled on the edge of my blanket.....and my FM caught it right away. In the wash it went and out came the disinfectant. Boy is that kitty in the proverbial doghouse!

I'm thankful for my warm "your bed" and keeping the hope going for all of the homeless.

Sweet warm dreams and mercy on those who don't have warmth and hope.

Just a footnote from mom here. Sandy continues to want to be hand fed and eats well when we do. She even has a special fork and a special place to try to sit when she gets her meals. It is so sweet, perhaps it is spoiling her but we want to keep her as happy and comfortable as a queen.

February 14, 2016

It was another double blanket day and even though it was below freezing, I went on a walk. My FPs are trying to make sure my hind leg muscles get worked. It's hard to be patient while I get stronger. The front part of my body wants to play with Annie and go after the ball but my hind part isn't moving along with the front very well. We are wondering if it will get better as my muscles develop. I can wag my tail but only a little so the physical therapy my FM does on me every day is supposed to loosen up the muscles and improve my circulation and gently stretch my spine. I don't like to have my tail messed with but I'm getting used to her rubbing it a little. It may be that my spine problem won't ever let me be very strong back there...waiting to see.

Happy Valentine's Day to the many fur babies and people who love me and I hope you know that you've made a huge impact on my life as well as the lives of so many others. Pass it on.

More from the same day:

My FPs send their love to all of my Valentines. I had a nice day and ate well and then was more playful than usual with Annie. I might get to meet the other three dogs in my family this week. Annie and Buddy know them really well and their names are Bella, Bucket, and Peter. I've figured out that my FPs are around them sometimes because I can sniff them when they get home and it's always the same smell. My poor FD says he doesn't know if he can handle having six dogs for the weekend...we will have to see.

All the four-legged people in my family are rescues...even the kitties. We are the best kind!!!! Snow tonight!

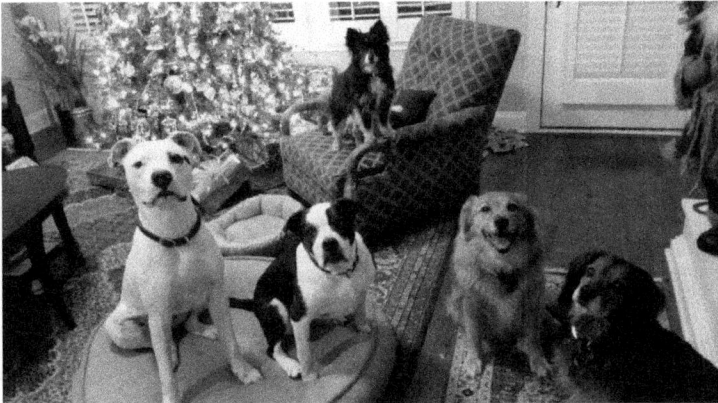

Left to Right: Peter (cousin), Bella (cousin) Bucket (cousin) Annie (sister) Buddy (brother)

February 16, 2016

All of you have been angels to me and I received this request from another rescue because of your kindness to me and how we all talk about paying it forward and how blessed I am. Just by sharing this on your pages we can all touch another one who needs all the healing and positive energy you can possibly send her. This must be part of the reason that I am being saved so I can help save others. But none of it would happen without each one of you who cares for me.

Thanks to you and your prayers, and the love of his family, Bozzie is healing well and walking on his own. Betty is going home tomorrow with a terminal diagnosis but a family who will make sure she is loved and nurtured every minute until she sees the Rainbow Bridge.

Please add this poor girl to your prayer list.

I did the BIG hill today. My FPs are determined to make my muscles work so I'll sleep like a log tonight. The weather was gloriously warm and I am hoping the cold days are gone for now!

Thank you. Thank you for your love, for your posts, for sharing and connecting the thousands of us who make a positive difference in this world. I love you.

From one of Sandy's Facebook friends:

Sandy, I have another angel that needs your prayers.. a girl named Curly that was brought in by kind strangers who found her on the side of a south Louisiana highway. She is at the vet's now getting fluids and nourishment. Her rescue group is **Tangi Humane Society**

Later on February 16

Icy day. FPs spent a lot of time making sure walkways and steps were cleared and safe for me. I did very well and have developed a new routine. I go every morning to my FMs side of the bed and somehow she knows I'm standing there because she awakens (at least enough to awaken my FP) and I get to go right outside. I got a massage by the fire in the fireplace and I actually enjoyed having my tail massaged. I walked better after it too!

I will be happy when warm weather comes and I can go outside without a blanket. I'm a sniffer and love to smell the grass but can't do it when it's covered in ice.

Please keep sending me the healing energy so my back legs get really strong and my spine allows me to trot and maybe even run one day.

Also, my FM has a dear friend whose fur baby is very sick. She is a white pit bull and the sweetest girl ever. Her name is Betty so please send healing energy and strength to her and her family.

Thank you for all you do for me.

Betty is a sweet pit mix that was rescued by Tuskegee veterinary student, Blair Anderson, now Dr. Blair Anderson, in Tallahassee, Florida. Betty has the funniest personality and lifts her head and turns it to the side when she wants to ignore you. She really got lucky to have Dr. Blair Anderson as a mom.

February 17, 2016

To so many of you who added Curly to your prayer list and who are watching her progress, my most sincere thank you!!!!

It was another BIG hill day and my FM tried walking all 3 of us together. After about a block she knew that was a poor decision on her part. Annie is the hard head in the bunch, Buddy is slow and steady and I am testing my independence by walking as far to the side as I can. As we were headed back, a lady with a Chow on a leash walked by us and Annie lost her mind. My FM says holding three leashes and three bags of poo was not fun so she told us we couldn't take walks together without our FD anymore.

The BIG hill is working my hind leg muscles and I guess that's going to be routine now since I've done it twice. And the other news is...there is this old chewed bone in the yard and it's been there since I got here. I've wanted to pick it up but it was sort of stuck and I didn't have strong enough paws to dig at it......until today and I GOT IT. And, I brought it in the house to show my FPs. They were so happy for me, even though the dirt was still falling off of it.

February 18, 2016

It was a BIG GLASS BOX day with a warm soapy massage, and I got a present in the mail (a Ginger Harness) for those awful nights when I am just so weak and my legs won't work on the steps to the back door. How nice to know I won't be skinning my legs on the brick steps anymore. The baths really still wear me out so we didn't do the BIG hill today. Will do it tomorrow.

The news about Curly is good. I've given my ok to them to post on my page so all of you who are pulling for her can stay updated. After all, isn't that what life is supposed to be... caring for others!

My love to all. I am still struggling with back legs so keep me in your hearts!

The ginger harness has saved my back! Sandy doesn't mind it at all and she seems almost happy to have us carry her hind end. We've decided we need dog ramps for her as it will help us and her on our icy steps. Kitty litter will be great for traction!

February 19 2016

Banner day! I used both hind legs to go up two steps!! And, I played catch with my FM and even retrieved the ball four times. Now, when I say "retrieved", I mean walked over and picked up. But even turning around has been a challenge so being willing to do it and go get the ball is a major deal here! I got lots of claps and "good girls." A small step for most but a giant one for me! In addition, I found a special rock in the yard and decided it needed to come in the house. My FPs picked it up and put it back in the yard but thanked me just the same. I'll get it tomorrow.

It seems for every really good day I follow it up with a hard day. My right hind leg just did not want to work today so my FM massaged and let me rest. She did walk me for a short bit so I don't get stiff. I loved being out in the yard and hope one day to be able to lie in the grass. My appetite wasn't quite up to par so I got extra goodies in it tonight to encourage me to eat it. I'd didn't eat it all but I did eat some.

Annie has taken to sleeping right beside me and I sort of like it. She knows her way around a food bowl and gets sort of pushy about my leftovers but FPs are onto her shenanigans.

I really like the weather being warmer and I didn't have to wear a coat at all today. Maybe by April it will stop being cold at all and I won't have to wear one for a while.

Special prayers tonight for all the dogs and cats who have had to have a leg amputated. I cannot imagine what that would be like and hope I never have to find out. But those that are tripods...they are brave souls and they are just on my mind tonight.

Some days we feel like it is one step forward and two steps back. Sandy is such a champion about trying, and she is also such a GSD! She is hard-headed and if she makes up her mind she's not doing it, she means it. It makes me laugh when she flat-out refuses to get up or eat. Her strong will is the only thing that kept her going through her neglect and abuse. I guess knowing that is why I laugh. Patience was never one of my virtues, so a life lesson for me is happening every day.

February 21, 2016

My FPs gave me the day off today. Annie and Buddy and I walked around in the yard a lot because it was a beautiful day. I ate well today and have had a nice afternoon nap. We will walk tomorrow I'm sure but today was rest. I don't know what it is about my food that Annie and Buddy are such thieves. If my FM turns her back they sneak ever so quietly to my bowl and eat. I have a habit of taking a mouthful and walking over onto the carpet to chew it up. My FM says to tell you that, yes, I have a rug to eat on but I choose to walk to the other rug. So while Annie is a pork chop and Buddy is a sausage, I am the one who needs to eat and gets the egg and coconut oil in my food. So my FM and FD have to decide how to re-locate my dishes and keep the thieves away.

My FC (foster cousin) Boz is doing well. His mom and dad used a Ginger Harness to help him for everything when he was first home from surgery, but now he only needs it on the ramp to the deck. He doesn't have to be contained anymore but isn't allowed to do stairs yet. So, since I have steps to get up (only three) to go out to the yard and back, my newest gadget (thanks to a very special friend of mine) is a Ginger Harness and it helps my legs greatly at the end of the day when I hurt and they aren't working very well. Boz is 125 pounds and a big gorgeous black and tan GSD so he makes me look small. He's also a very sweet baby and adored at home. Actually, he and his sister Maggie (RIP BEAUTIFUL GIRL!) are the reason I have my FPs. And all of this, my rescue, started because of them.

So here I am, lying by the fire, with a bed in the den and a bed in the master bedroom. I get a bath every 3 days, I have regular meals, I have treats and supplements and coats and toys and blankets and Annie and Buddy and my kitties, my FPs, and most of all, I have all of you. You all keep my FPs inspired to keep on helping me and you inspire me to keep taking one step at a time.

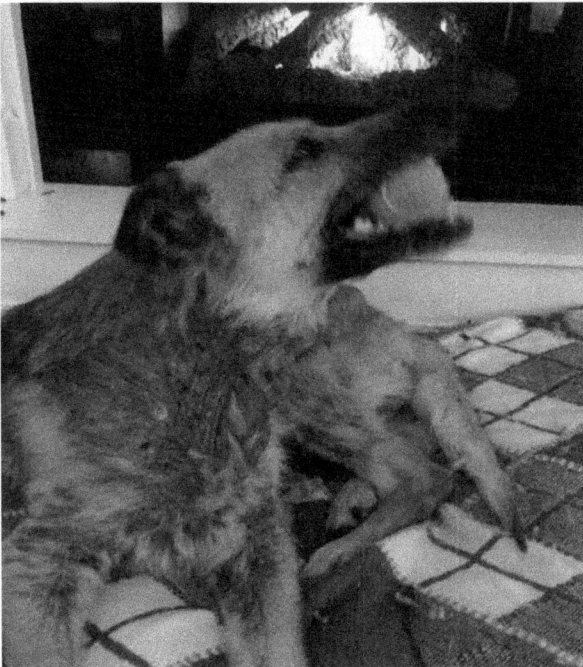

February 22 2016

My FM had the blessing of holding and feeding and loving some of the Vicktory Dogs at Best Friends Animal Sanctuary in Utah. Being a Virginian, she has a special goal to help people understand about this horrifying event and the saving of these dogs. So, because she is an FM who believes this is her purpose in life, she asks you to look at their website and support the movie touring the country: www.bestfriends.org

I do so hate that buzzy thing but my FM made me be still to do my front feet. I was limping because my nails needed the buzzy thing and I had run away from her twice earlier this past weekend but today, she won. And now I'm not limping. So she won. I got a wonderful visit today from my rescuer and my massage therapist. I am actually pretty active tonight and feeling better. I still hate the buzzy thing. And I've found out that if I turn my nose up at the food without any special things in it, I can get my FPs to add some very good things.

So here is a post on that pitiful girl I shared last week, Curly. She's not thriving very well so needs all the prayers and positive healing energy you can possibly send her. The power that all of you have just by doing this is beyond your wildest imagination. I am proof.

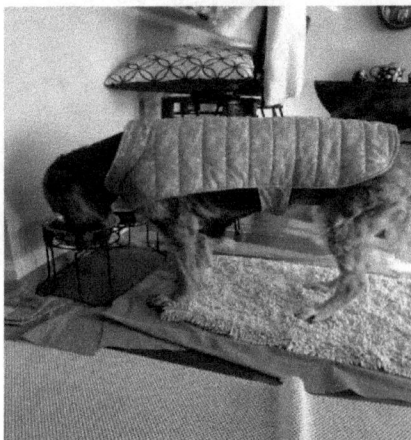

Later from the same day

From her rescue: Curly is doing well this morning. She did not eat very well over the weekend but is doing much better today. She is drinking a little on her own. The transfusion did get her blood count up, but still not in the normal range. Dr. Toney is doing some more bloodwork today and will be sending it to the lab to make sure there is nothing else going on. Curly is moving around a little bit but is still not able to stand or sit up at this point. She has a friend that visits with her daily, and between pets and loving, "they" do "Words with Friends." Thanks for all the prayers and donations, we still have a long way to go, and our bill is already $1,000.00; we could not continue her care without the continued support of so many who already have fallen in love with her. Please continue to share and support Curly, because her battle is not over. Thanks again for everyone's love, thoughts and support in saving our sweet girl Curly!

February 23, 2016

I am a picky picky eater. One day I like my food, the next day I don't. Keeps my FPs guessing and today they finally resorted to wild boar with no grain. Now my FM doesn't know if I just ate it because I was hungry or because I like it. Ha ha. She doesn't think it's funny.

We now have a toy bin. I guess all of them lying around was driving my FPS crazy. But Buddy picks them up one at a time and carries them to his own little pile in the dining room. My FD has to go pick them up and put them away every night!

I have a little fuzz on one side of my bare back and my saddle is filling in. Tomorrow is big glass box day again. We didn't walk today because of the rain.

I'm so thankful for all the people who love me. I'm so thankful that it helps my FPs know there really are good people in this world...they just don't get the attention all the horrible people do.

I also heard there is a dog meat trade in Southeast Asia....that is so sickening. **Soi Foundation** is trying to save a lot of them. Please remind your friends and loved ones to adopt, sponsor or foster...it's pretty easy with social media these days.

February 24, 2016

Hiding in a closet with FPs, Annie, Buddy, Tipper and Lulu was not my fave thing to do, plus I had to share a bed with Annie and that wasn't fun either. Those flat ringing things my FPs talk to kept sounding an alarm and my FP kept looking at it. My FM sat on the floor and the stupid cat (Tipper) curled up and went to sleep on her lap like nothing was amiss. We had something called a "tornado" warning and the storm was right on us. Buddy did not want to go in the closet so we all got bribed with treats. Before we went in the closet, the wind was so strong it shook the windows and the wind chimes were flipping all around. Lightning came and water was coming down in sheets from the sky. Everything turned dark outside and the alarms kept going off so we went in the closet. I wanted to come out because I knew my FM had just mixed up a big meatloaf and it was sitting on the counter ready for the oven. Side note: I didn't get any.

It was a scary stormy afternoon and evening but we are all safe and nothing harmed. (Except maybe my dignity from sharing a bed with Miss Porky Chop Annie).

Using the buzzy thing has become a NO-NO with me so my FM gave up and will let the vet handle it.

Hope all of you are safe and warm and dry tonight.

Later the same day

*"All things bright and beautiful, all things great and small, all things
wise and wonderful, our Father made them all. "*

Run sweet Curly girl. Run free, run healthy, run feeling no pain, and
knowing you are loved and we hurt for the pain you suffered at the
hands of humans. May the heavens that sent you receive you into the
infinity that will hold all souls in love and kindness.

Love,

Sandy, FPs, Annie, Buddy, Tipper and Lulu

From Curly's friend:

*RIP Curly . . . Thank you to everyone for their prayers and
donations to try to save her. She passed early this morning. (I had not
received the news prior to my earlier post.) Please give your own fur
babies a hug, and Sandy, you keep up the good fight!!*

February 25, 2016

My FM does not like politics because she says it makes her head hurt.
Something called "Republicans and Democrats" keeps coming on that
thing over the fireplace that talks and while my FD watches, my FM
uses her laptop. Just think if all the money spent on debates and
campaigns was spent to rescue and take care of homeless and abused
and neglected fur babies. If that were to happen there wouldn't be any
one of us without a roof over our heads, food to eat, and loving hands
to soothe us. Can you imagine?

"You can say that I'm a dreamer. But I'm not the only one."

~ John Lennon

February 26, 2016

I've been a bit off today. Not much appetite until tonight. I was limping around more than usual and I had run away from the buzzy thing so many times that my FM gave up. But, she remembered she has dog nail trimmers so she used them and I didn't mind. So she trimmed my nails and, voila! I am not limping as much. She was right! My feet were hurting me. So I ate my dinner and am enjoying the fire in the fireplace.

Southeast German Shepherd Rescue is so good at making sure I get the medicine and vitamins and treats that all their pups get and I think there have been two more dogs fostered because of my story. People far and wide continue to send me their love and I want all of you to know how thankful I am for the healing energies and positive encouragement you have sent my way. I have a little ridge of hair down my spine and my tummy is almost all pink. By April I might get to go to one bath a week as my skin clears up. The nerve damage in my back is always going to be there but as I get stronger muscles it will help.

February 27, 2016

We have had a couple of very gloomy wet days and mom thinks maybe that's why I'm not up to par. I have had more trouble getting around the past few days and my front feet have begun to sort of paddle when I walk. I can't walk in a straight line because my back end is so weak on the right side and intend to move more towards the left. We have Dr. Ruth coming on Tuesday so mom and dad will see what she thinks. I've been very fussy in the evenings and we haven't been able to walk because of the weather. Mom will talk to Dr. Ruth about my anxiety too. I did play ball with mom early this afternoon...I lie there and she throws it so I can catch it. She gets more exercise than I do because although I am pretty good at catching, I can't move much while lying down so she's the retriever. Mom and dad are huge believers in the quality of life and they watch mine very closely.

Tonight in our area, two beautiful huskies are missing and feared stolen. We are praying for their safe return.

If you see something, say something. It applies to animals too!

February 29, 2016

Having a wonderful warm day and going to walk the big hill! Can't wait for spring to be able to try to lie down in the warm dry grass!

March 1, 2016

My FM's heart hurts tonight because her good friend's pittie died suddenly today. Her name was Betty and her mom is a veterinarian. Betty was rescued by her mom when her mom was in vet school. She was a white pittie and only 10 years old. Please keep her mom and dad and brother in your prayers and send them the healing energies all of you have within you and have shared with me. My FM believes that our energies live beyond our physical bodies and knows there is a Rainbow Bridge where we transition into happy healthy beings.

I am doing ok. Bit by bit and hair by hair. I'm such a sloppy drinker that my FPs have moved my bowls into the master bathroom on the tile floor so that's taking some getting used to. Also if any of you know a kind of bowl that works for a long-nosed GS like me, could you let me know. I lick my food to the side of my bowl and then if it's hard to get out, I won't eat it. Then my FPs have to get a big spoon and stir it and yes, they spoon-feed me. I like it that way but I think they are wanting me to eat all on my own.

Thank you and prayers for Betty's people.

Yes, she's learned that the big spoon comes to her aid to get the last morsels that she licks into the edge of her bowl. She sits there with begging eyes that melt your heart, and even though it spoils her, she can have as many big spoonsful as she wants!

March 2, 2016

No worries my sweet friends. I am doing ok. I think better than a couple of days ago. Nothing major happening here except my FM moved my bowls to the master bath and since the big glass box is in there, I found it a bit alarming and didn't want to go in there at first. But Annie and Buddy eat in the laundry room which is tiled and there isn't room for me and them too. So since the master bath is large, my FM put my bowls in there on the tile floor. I am a hugely sloppy water slurper, and the hardwood was at risk where I was when I was so weak. But now with a bath rug and tile floor my drips won't be bad. I got used to it (sort of) today. And I've switched to eating only dry food not mixed with wet and I think I like it better.

My progress is huge compared to 8 weeks ago! I'll need supplements and vitamins for a long time, probably the rest of my life, but that's ok because I like life now, and count on my Facebook Family because I know they love me.

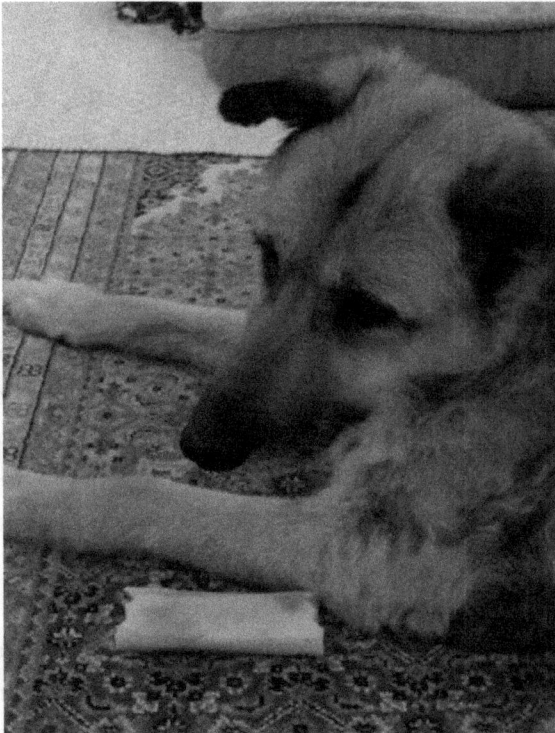

March 3, 2016

Look at my happy self! I did the big hill yesterday and today! I got half the dose of pain meds and I am better today than ever. Go figure! My FM plays catch with me (I LOVE a tennis ball)! I don't retrieve very well but I can flat snatch a ball out of the air if it's thrown within my range of movement!

Please keep the prayers and healing spirits coming here! They are working pure miracles for a crippled neglected starved girl who is experiencing it firsthand. HIS eye is on the sparrow!

March 4, 2016

Guess what I got today! And right in time! I take vitamins with antioxidants and Coseguin and this! Of course coconut oil and peanut butter are part of my diet too plus eggs. Thank you my sweet friends!

March 5, 2016

I've had a day of rest and tonight got up off of my "your bed", walked over to the tennis ball, and took it to my FD! I can catch it if it's a short throw! And I wagged my tail when my FM told me what a good girl I am! I've gotten used to the change of location for my water bowl; however, I like my food in the bowl on the floor while I lie down. I pick at it, nibble, then get up and move then go back and nibble then take another break. Last night Lulu stuck her nose in my dish and I woofed at her to get away. My FPs laughed. Then today Annie stuck her nose in MY bowl and I woofed at her. She started to get snarky so my FM shooed her away. I'm pretty sure Annie was surprised I stood my ground. So everyone is winding down for a long cold night. Here are pictures of Tipper and Lulu and Annie and Buddy.

March 6 2016

My rescue organization is in the process of trying to rescue several GS dogs from horrible situations. In order to pull a dog from a shelter, **Southeast German Shepherd Rescue** must have a foster spot available who is approved by them. That means that there is a time period to get approved as a foster so you can be approved and ready for that call in the night when a raid on a puppy mill happens or when law enforcement finds a dog in need or when a dog is a day away from being euthanized in a kill shelter. I was rescued two days before my scheduled death by someone who absolutely trusted she could find a foster immediately. So, if you've ever considered being a foster, let the rescue organization of your choice know so they have a soft place to land when things start falling apart at a rapid pace. Dog rescues often happen in the dead of night, on a lonely road, an abandoned home or farm, a high-kill shelter, and even in a courtroom. SGSR has to be ready and I hope if you can help them be ready to pull dogs in need you will check the box that you are willing to foster.

My love to all of you. I am one of the lucky ones.

We never thought of ourselves as potential fosters to a dog. Maybe that's why Sandy got dropped in our lives so urgently, and we were taught that making room for one more was not really a big deal. She is the most amazing, trusting, gentle creature. I often wonder how she could ever trust a human being again. The lesson is ours to learn.

March 8, 2016

I've had a tough two days. I didn't do well on my walk yesterday so my FM made it short. We walked the big hill today and I was with my FD. Annie and Buddy were with my FM. I just gave up a block from home and sat down then lay down on the grass. My FM hurried home to get my Ginger Harness but I did get up and go a bit further. I was exhausted so I got the water served to me while I panted on my to "your bed". I slept all afternoon and ate a good dinner. Am resting with my FD while my FM is at a rehearsal. It may be time for more Tramadol. I'm getting Rimadyl but two days of backsliding are worrisome. Send prayers.

March 9, 2016

Today I rested. Tomorrow I get more meds. I ate well but I'm not much on moving around. My FPs are looking into water therapy and further treatments and checking to see if Southeast German Shepherd Rescue will help with the treatments if there are any. I'll keep you all posted on how I feel with meds. Thank you from the bottom of my heart for your healing energy and prayers. My FPs thank you too and we know your support has been so wonderful. My cup is half full because although I am having trouble walking, I have soft beds and comfy blankets, supplements and good food, I don't itch anymore and I know I am loved.

March 10, 2016

There is no way to explain the power of your positive healing thoughts and your prayers. My FD gave me a total body massage today and I proceeded to get up, try to get Annie to play with me, met my FM at the door with my tail wagging and had not had a bit of Tramadol yet. I am perky and ate a full dinner. I did get the medicine and am watching every move my FPs are making. It's pretty obvious that I feel better! We will take it very slowly on the walking thing but I have a marked improvement over the past three days! Every one of your messages gets read, every person who likes my page is appreciated, every prayer loved and every day a reason to be thankful for all and each of you.

It is so interesting to watch how the typical German Shepherd characteristics begin to show up as Sandy's health stabilizes. She never takes her eyes off of us as we move around the den and kitchen. She is on point mentally, even though her poor body is betraying her. Her personality has slowly shown up, and she is one sassy little girl when she feels good. She is a quick study and has figured out how to "invite" Annie or the cats over for a head rub if she wants one. She reads off of us so well that we have to be very careful about showing concern.

March 11, 2016

My FM promises that she will take more pictures and videos tomorrow. I had a good day, got my visit to the big glass box, had a full massage, and a visit from my Southeast German Shepherd Rescue angel. And I EVEN WENT UP TWO STEPS BY MYSELF VOLUNTARILY AND DOWN TWO!

All of you are my angels who love me and pray for me. My FPs think that the reason I've done so well is because of all the healing wishes that create the energies that connect with my spirit. So please know how much we all appreciate what you do in sending us love and prayers. Bless the beasts and the children...you are their voice.

March 12, 2016

I witnessed a miracle today! Foster cousin Boz, who is well now, came to our house to meet his new sister, Sierra, a beautiful German Shepherd from **Southeast German Shepherd Rescue**. Sierra's FM, Susan, brought her to our house to meet Boz. Susan has nursed Sierra back to health from surgery after numerous malignant tumors were removed from her breasts after being neglected by a former owner. She came to Susan just after surgery and required major care of drainage tubes and sutures. She is a beauty now and my heart goes out to her FM for the empty space she must feel in her house. But, Sierra has gone to my Foster Aunt and Uncle where all creatures live with absolute love in a gorgeous fenced yard. She will be treated like the miracle she is and loved beyond measure. I took a walk today after they left and have been a really happy girl.

I received the best present today for my FPs to use when I come in with wet feet or when I get rain on my head. The cutest towels with little pockets for my FPs hands.

Thanks to all of you for being part of my world and my miracles!

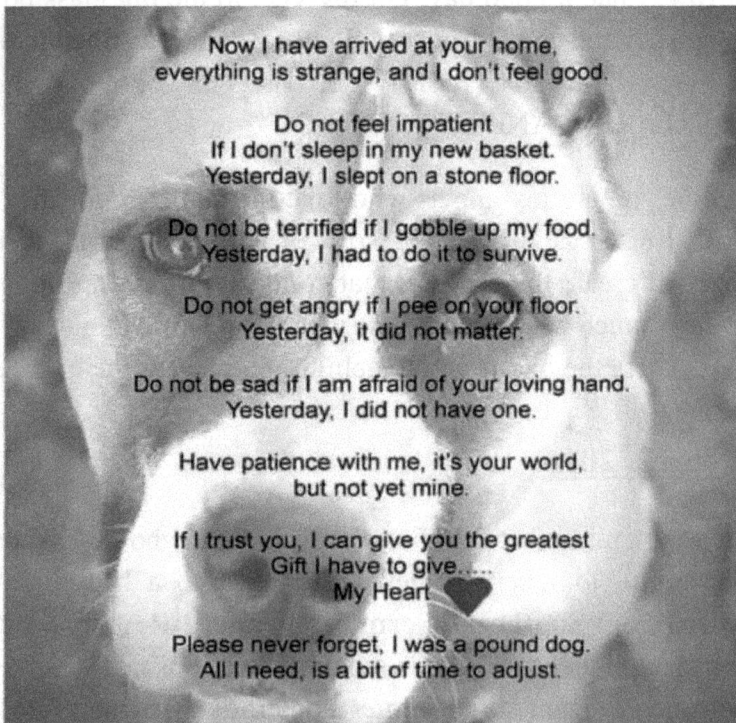

Now I have arrived at your home,
everything is strange, and I don't feel good.

Do not feel impatient
If I don't sleep in my new basket.
Yesterday, I slept on a stone floor.

Do not be terrified if I gobble up my food.
Yesterday, I had to do it to survive.

Do not get angry if I pee on your floor.
Yesterday, it did not matter.

Do not be sad if I am afraid of your loving hand.
Yesterday, I did not have one.

Have patience with me, it's your world,
but not yet mine.

If I trust you, I can give you the greatest
Gift I have to give......
My Heart

Please never forget, I was a pound dog.
All I need, is a bit of time to adjust.

March 13, 2016

It is a dark and stormy night. A lazy Sunday of being in the yard, a short walk and back curled up on my "your bed". Tomorrow will begin a week of hunting for the right kind of therapy for me. And the right place to get it. Will be reaching out to you my friends once I have more good info about it.

March 14, 2016

Got some new traction boots today and got bribed to try them out on the hardwood floors. I'm not sure about them yet, but I have a feeling I'll be styling these boots pretty frequently. Love and licks to my friends who sent them!!!!

I ate very well today since it was mostly canned food. Crunch food is now not my favorite so my FM wants the vet to look at my teeth! Lots of getting checked on all the time.

Little Miss Sandy has decided to be picky about her food now that she is not starving. Looks like we will be mixing dry food with wet food. And, by the way, she has us very well trained to feed her with a fork. Every single bite! If we put the bowl in front of her, she looks up at us like we have three eyes as if to say, "What's wrong with you? Don't you know how to pick up a fork?" Oh yes, the boots. Well, she also decided to refuse to get up once we put them on her feet.

March 15, 2016

My FM promises a picture of me and my boots tomorrow! We are working our way through all the medical references and will be scheduling some therapy soon. I am eating well and loving the good weather BUT I did NOT like the last two nights of horrible booming thunder, hail, and frog-strangling rain. All five of us were huddled under my FPs legs trying to hide from the flashes of light and the booming. If God was moving the furniture around last night, HE sure was dropping a lot of it! I got a really good massage today and walked a longer way than I have since my setback. There's a really silly Cane Corso next door who woofs me at the fence every day and then when I walk up to the fence he runs away. The black Lab next door is a good friend and we like to rub noses. I love the attention I am getting and am now comfortable lying on the rug and don't have to use my "your bed" all the time. My back right leg is the one I drag a bit so I have some spinal issues that we are hoping will improve with more muscle tone. It's been 8 weeks since I was rescued so I've come a long way since then! Thanks and love to all of you!!!

March 16, 2016

Prayers. Sometimes, in fact often times, when prayers are offered on social media my FPs and other people read it, are thankful for the moment, and then get rushed into their daily business or nightly routines, forgetting ..., forgetting the power in each of you who has offered prayers, who has sent healing energy and positive life-giving thoughts my way.

How odd, that people seem to only understand this power in compartmentalized moments. Perhaps the love of a dog can teach humans the continuum of prayer, the power of healing through the energy you each create. To see, to experience the miracle of moving towards health and happiness and pure contentment by seeing a dog like me able to walk again, able to ask for a head rub or nudge Annie or Buddy to attempt a playful act, to watch me fast asleep with an almost full coat after healing from mange, is almost unbelievable. And so I am a result of the healing energies, of the power of the prayers and the love sent to me.

My prayers are never compartmentalized. I love giving unconditional love and looking forward with hope every waking minute. Thank you my friends!

Love to all of you!

I have come to believe that loving an animal is the closest thing I will know to divine power. The experience is all-consuming and passionate yet, different than loving one's own child. Perhaps it is because the animals have no voice but ours.

March 18, 2016

Well my FM is busy busy and my FD is busy busy. We have my FC's here .... Bella, Peter, and Bucket so there are 6 of us plus 2 kitties. They will be here until Sunday so there's been very little alone time. I did get a nice massage today and am actively making sure no one else eats my food or lies down at my FP's feet.

Stay posted this weekend for updates on my FM's relentless work to obtain my medical records as it hasn't proved to be an easy task. Seems the X-rays done at the shelter that had me originally won't be released to my FM and we may have to get new ones.

March 20, 2016

Enjoying the quiet of just us three but have to say that having Peter, Bella and Bucket was an inspiration for me to move around more and eat all of my food and not be so picky. They are such good babies and my FM and FD were quite good with six of us.

The kitties have reappeared since they like to be mysteriously gone when the 6 of us are here. I suspect they were staying upstairs to keep Peter and Bella from chasing them.

My FM is still working on getting all my records so we can go see another vet for second opinion (or first opinion depending on how you look at it). Her plan is to keep all of you aware of how this goes since it's been a bit bumpy so far.

My love and thanks to all of you for thinking of me and I want you to know I only have the lower part of my back that is still bare. My fur is coming in nicely and thanks to all the vitamins and supplements you all have sent my FF believes it is key to my progress. I've been here two months and the transformation is amazing!

<u>March 21, 2016</u>

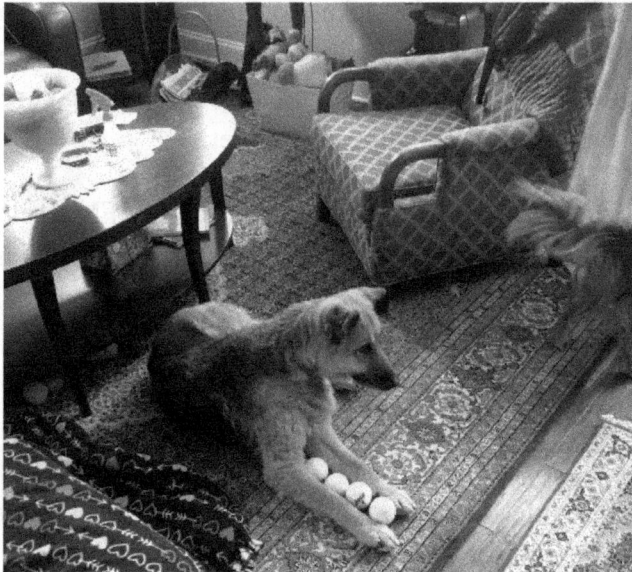

Here I am next to my "your bed". I have my balls lined up to keep Annie from getthing them

March 23, 2016

I'm doing ok! Back legs are a tad stronger every day but my spinal issues are the same. But, my "your bed" is comfy, my tummy is full, and tomorrow is big glass box day. I love my tennis ball and my blankets; I love my FPs and my Annie, Buddy and Tipper and Lulu! I ventured into the kitchen tonight for treats and am getting used to my boots. I don't slip with them on but apparently I look like a ballerina with tap shoes because my FM says I'm silly about them.

All of us are sending love to those affected by the ISIS terrorist bombing today. Those of us who have suffered at the hands of cruelty understand how it hurts and depend on people like all of you to care for others.

Nice weather, and ate a big dinner...more pics and posts as the weekend gets here. My FD will try to remember to take pics on our walk tomorrow.

Watching Sandy walk in her boots was hilarious. She picked her feet up like a Tennessee Walking Horse, and looked like a young colt trying to stand for the first time. We had to laugh even though we felt sorry for her. These boots will be a lifesaver to keep her steady and protect the feet where she seems to have no feeling.

March 25, 2016

Good news! Getting vet records! Now if we can only get the shelter records! Going to my FPs vet next week for a thorough check. By the way, I ate 4 1/2 cups of food today! Every improvement seems to excite my FPs and I have pretty much decided that I am a part of this family and I like it that way! I got brushed today because I am actually shedding. Hard to believe since I had no hair when I got here.

Look what I got today from one of my sweet friends! The Easter Bunny came early!

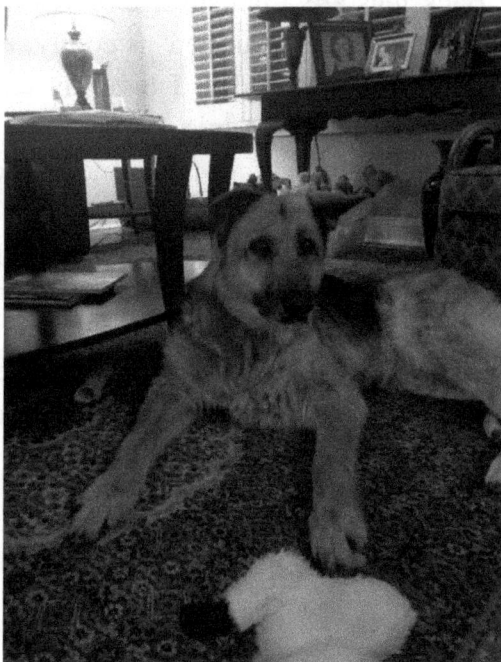

The tradition of Easter means love lives, living our life should be based on love...... Love is saving me.

March 26, 2016

In the past few days my ability to walk has diminished and today has been pretty bad. My FPs are watching me carefully and making sure to pick me up so I don't drag my hind legs when trying to walk. I need many prayers and powerful healing sent my way and please send some strength and wisdom to my FPs right now. I will see a vet on Monday. I am not in pain, just frustrated that I can't move around. My FPs are cutting back on my food intake because I can't support myself but will do it in a healthy managed way.

Thank you for the love you continue to send our way.

This is such a roller coaster ride. Two or three days will be good and then a bad one which is worse than the last bad one. We are beginning to teach ourselves the inevitability of this horrible disease, and still hoping this will be the breakthrough, that all we are doing will be the key to finding a cure for this disease. I take some solace in knowing that, at the very least, we are educating people about this disease called Degenerative Myelopathy in dogs.

We are becoming more aware that Sandy's life, her story, may be the one thing that makes a difference to even one dog.

March 27, 2016

Easter Blessings and love to all of you. I have had a quiet day and still having great difficulty walking. I have made it with help to the yard thanks to my Ginger Harness and my appetite is still good. My FPs will get me to the vet asap. Providing ownership complications don't arise, they want to try to get me referred **to North Carolina State Veterinary Clinic** if at all possible for options but the vet has to refer me. Timing is of the essence because my rescue organization is not financially able to go for extensive treatments for dogs like me, so if all falls into place, my fosters can adopt me and choose their own path to treat me which is what I'm hoping for. I get all sorts of supplements and joint supplements but I have a spine issue that is affecting how my legs can move. My FPs are taking extra care to help me and promise to keep all of you aware of the situation. The front part of me is so happy and I am feeling so much better about life but my back end isn't cooperating.

The blessing in all of this is the love you have demonstrated for me. We usually try to "like" every comment on my page so forgive my FM if that doesn't happen today. Please know we will read every one of them!

We know you will all be with us on this journey!

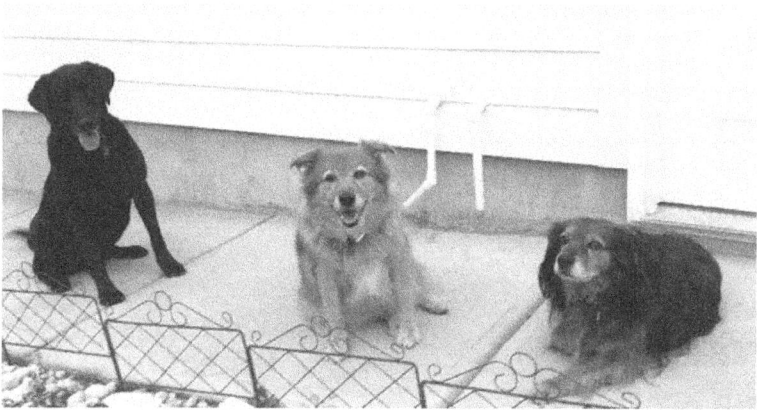

My next-door neighbor, Cash with Annie and Buddy

The Learning

March 28, 2016

Well, my vet went over me with a fine-toothed comb and the news is not good. He reviewed all of the records that the rescue organization sent to us. I exhibit all symptoms of DM (Degenerative Myelopathy) and he is 97% sure of this diagnosis. Even if it was spine and disc problem, which he believes it is not, I am not a candidate for surgery due to my traumatic history. He will refer us to **North Carolina State School of Veterinary Medicine** if we like but feels sure that all that can be done now is palliative care. He recommends we add gabapentin to my meds. He estimates I will lose all use of my rear legs in 3 to 4 months.

We will continue with the 75 mg of Rimadyl twice a day and 100 mg of Tramadol twice a day.

In light of his diagnosis, my FPs will continue to love me and keep me comfortable and well-nourished and safe, and promise to make decisions based on my comfort and quality of life.

I am sure you understand, as they consider me a part of the family already. I am beyond grateful for all the love and prayers you have sent. Please keep all of us in your hearts as we continue on my journey. My FPs say I am a blessing to them and that my desire to survive and live is beyond measure. In the days to follow I will keep you posted on how I am doing. Remember to hug your fur babies extra tightly tonight, linger a moment over them to say goodnight, and greet them in the morning with a smile, a gentle rub, and a ton of patience.

March 29, 2016

Thank each and every one of you for your kind words, prayers, offers, and loyalty. My FPs are working on ways to determine what our next steps are. If any of you has experience with hydrotherapy and acupuncture please advise on what to expect in expenses to do this. I've been very happy today and even though I fall a lot, I am still determined to move around. We are looking at beneficial foods and received an incredible offer of wheels from Max, a GS who was also a therapy dog at St. Jude's! What an honor to be given this incredibly generous gift!

You know, I already take a supplement called DGP that has Feverfew extract and Turmeric (one of my kind FB friends sent a bottle), I get fish oil, Dasaquin, and a super vitamin with A, D, B12 and E (which also came from a FB friend). And I get a fatty acid complex called EFAC. My FPs plan to continue on this regimen unless while learning more about DM they find out it isn't good for me.

So many of you have sent me good things to recover from my neglect and starvation and now they will hopefully keep me happy and as healthy as possible in this journey.

We have some hurdles to cross before I know for sure about my therapy and possible adoption. You all have no idea how much strength you give my FPs and especially my FM. You lift us up, and we are ever thankful.

We hated this news. So, we had a decision to make about what to think of it all. We have chosen to make Sandy's life significant, to let her teach us the joy in every achievement, no matter how small. We know she was sent to us for a reason and that her life has a purpose. The reality is that we know in our hearts she is ours.

March 30, 2016

I am proud to tell you that I now have a mom and dad and no more foster parents! I am officially a member of the household now, and my parents are relieved that they will be able to make all the decisions concerning my well-being. It is a bit overwhelming for them but now I have a brother and a sister and real cousins! Boz and his new sister Pearl, Peter and Bella and Bucket...we are all family now!

So many of you have asked me to start a GoFundMe page so stay tuned because my mom is going to look into it so I can get acupuncture and hydrotherapy to see if it helps at all.

Each one of YOU has been an inspiration to my folks to keep pushing and keep trying and to keep on with all of my needs. Blessings have flowed to me and I have all of you to thank.

I will continue to post so you can keep up with me through this journey. Perhaps I can be a voice for all the dogs with DM. My mom is pretty persistent so I suspect she'll become the resident expert here on DM. Please continue to hold me in your hearts and pray for me. Send healing and light but also pray for the thousands of pups who are still in cages awaiting someone to love them, or chained in a bare yard, or crouching behind trash cans scavenging for food. I really am one of the lucky ones.

Stay tuned!

It could not be any other way. This sweet girl has come to trust us and know she is safe. She knows she is a priority with us and that her "your bed" is, indeed, hers. She has nurtured us with her spirit of determination, she is teaching us boundless patience, and she loves us with abandon. We have realized that the blessing in all of this journey is what she is showing us and teaching us, not what we are doing for her. Her spirit has reached into our hearts and bound us together.

March 31

This is my mom and dad! Thought you'd like to see them. Dad's name is Michael and Mom's name is Diana. OUR last name is Mahoney!!!!!!

Where to start and what to say? How do I even begin to tell all of you what hope I have? How do I thank all of you for the love and support? Even my Mom doesn't know! We have been so overwhelmed ever day by the prayers and healing and love sent our way, and now, I am actually being referred to North Carolina State School of Veterinary Medicine for a full evaluation and therapy. Not only will I be able to do this because of you but I will be able to get acupuncture and massage therapy. For a 10-year-old GS who never even had enough to eat, who never had a bed, and who only dreamt of never being cold, it is all hard to take in.

My mom and dad want to assure everyone that my fund will only go to help me, and they are opening a separate bank account strictly for me. Every time I see a doctor or get a therapy I will share it with you, my FB family.

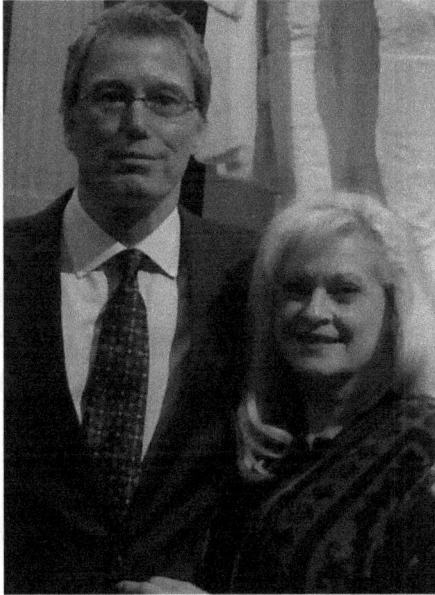

Michael and Diana

Each of you matters to us. Your kindness and strength have helped us more than you know. In the days to come, we will be helping Sandy to compensate for her back legs when she can, we will love her unconditionally, we will spoil her rotten, and we will seek the very best treatment to make her happy and live a life of good things. We count on you to follow Sandy's journey, and we'd like to try to increase awareness about degenerative myelopathy. Thank you for walking with us!

April 1, 2016

We have an APPOINTMENT at **North Carolina State Veterinary Clinic**!! It is on May 9, so we have a way to go but we are on their call list if they get a cancellation beforehand. And, I have my own bank account. My mom and dad opened an account just for my GoFundMe funds so every penny will be spent on my healthcare.

It was warm out today and I got impatient with waiting for my mom and dad to help me up the two steps to the back stoop, so I did it on my own, hopping like a rabbit with my hind legs.

My mom thinks the gabapentin might be affecting my appetite, so she's cutting back tonight to see how hungry I am in the morning.

And, there's an underwater hydrotherapy tub at the dog spa right around the corner!!!! So, my mom will talk to our vet in the morning to see if I should go ahead or if I should wait until after the May appointment.

My enormous thanks to all of you again for all you have done and continue to do for me. If anyone decides they need to know how to access my Go Fund Me account, it is in one of my posts earlier this week.

With love from all of us!

April 3, 2016

I received good news that my wheels from Max are on the way! It's good timing because I've begun sort of hopping around and occasionally just dragging my hind end. I'm still able to go potty but this morning needed help standing for the first time. I'm so glad I have a mom and dad to help me and can't imagine dogs suffering from DM without help. There is a blood test now to check for it according to my Mom's research. She's going to post some things later on today about signs of this disease.

I am alert and working on being totally relaxed. My front end stays tense and tired because I'm doing all the work with my shoulders and front legs. It's a bit cool today outside so we are staying in, since cold is probably not great for me at this point. I still have one big patch on my hind end that is bare. Working on those little hairlettes!

Ok, here is a beginning of helping everyone understand DM. Hope these tidbits of info help you and others know a bit more and it sure is helping my family

What causes degenerative myelopathy?

Degenerative myelopathy is associated with a genetic abnormality in dogs. The most common form is due to a genetic mutation in a gene coding for superoxide dismutase, a protein responsible for destroying free radicals in the body. Free radicals are part of the natural defense mechanism but become harmful when they are produced in excessive quantities causing cell death and a variety of degenerative diseases. The same gene mutation can also cause a form of motor neuron disease in humans, and is similar to Lou Gehrig's Disease or ALS.

I've not had a good day but my mom is moving quickly for tomorrow on the acupuncture and water therapy. My friends, you keep us inspired and it's not about the fund. It's about how we are all part of each other; we are all part of the universal energies and are bound by unbreakable bonds. You are all part of our hearts and each time you visit my page or send me encouragement we are lifted up. Isn't that what we are all here to learn how to do? To lift each being up, to end suffering and to be kind and merciful. That's the goal. My spirit is lifted by each of you.

April 4, 2016

We are on the way to North Carolina State vet school emergency. Sandy isn't able to stand or walk, so we will let you know. It's 4:45 Daylight Savings Time in North Carolina.

We are still at North Carolina State Veterinary Clinic ER. Tests and X-rays and neurology consultation. Thank you for all the prayers; it lifts our spirits! Knowing she is back with the doctors and wondering if she's been abandoned again is killing me, but we know this is where she must be right now.

Finally, on the way home, X-rays of the spine are just horrendous. The nightmare this poor baby has lived through! We have narrowed it down to two problems, degenerative disc disease and DM, but we will have definitive DM results in two weeks. It could be a cancerous mass on the spine, but we wouldn't know unless we did MRI. And treatment would be the same, considering her health and age. So, we will keep her on anti-inflammatory meds and pain meds. Have to order special shoes to protect her feet all the time. Will proceed with hydrotherapy and acupuncture. Thank you; we cannot begin to say what we feel for your love and support.

I am a worn-out girl. Mom and Dad have decided I need a day of rest so acupuncture and hydrotherapy will be on Wednesday or Thursday. Many heartfelt thanks for your prayers, for the healing energy I will continue to need, and for the love.

Elizabeth Massie is an author and poet who went to high school with my mom.

*Here are her words from her book "**Night Benedictions**" that say everything we want to say:*

"Night 232. Darkness hides only that which is seen by the eyes, while those things that are seen by the soul need no light. Love lives on throughout the brilliant day and across the reach of the deepest night, unfazed, unfettered. The sun will rise and set, the stars will shine then retreat. Life will begin and end. But love that we give freely

will always be remembered; and love we receive will be with us into eternity."

Elizabeth Massie

April 5, 2016

My mom and dad decided I needed to rest today and that I've been too stressed by all the activity yesterday so my appointment for acupuncture and hydrotherapy and physical therapy will be on Friday. I've done really well with being held up by the harness and even late today was moving my back feet as if walking on them but the harness had all the weight. I still squat but they hold me up. I've eaten two really good meals today and even growled at Annie when she came too close to my dinner bowl! It made my mom and dad laugh. I love being rubbed so hopefully my PT session will be soothing. My folks will be there to make sure I know I'm ok.

If you have a dog who has DM, please be sure to let us know so we can include you in our prayers!

April 7, 2016

It is a miracle even if for a day! I stood on my own and walked around the den most of the afternoon and evening. My mom and dad were flabbergasted! I was one happy girl! I even went to the toy box and dug out a toy I wanted! I've learned to whine for attention so my mom or dad rubs me when I whine. I'm tired tonight but it was pretty wonderful to stand on my own legs and walk to the door to greet my mom! Happy day here and we are over the moon thankful for today. Tomorrow is a big whopper of a day with hydrotherapy and acupuncture. Annie and Buddy are riding in the car with me to keep me from being anxious. I like it when they are along!

Mom found this on the web...... Reading stuff all the time to learn more. All of the info below is from the website of S.F. Chapman, DVM, who also believes in a holistic veterinary approach.

The acknowledged veterinary expert on Degenerative Myelopathy of German Shepherds is Dr. R. M. Clemmons at the University of Florida. He has been studying DM in Shepherds for years: DM Study His website is a gold mine of information about this disease. One apparent omission on the site is any mention of the genetic testing for the SOD 1 mutation.

I attended Dr. Clemmons's Degenerative Myelopathy lecture at the American Holistic Veterinary Medical conference in Kansas City last month, where he discussed diagnosis and treatment of DM. I asked him what role DM testing for the SOD 1 mutation should have in diagnosis of the disease and in breeding programmes. He said that the current SOD 1 DM test is not useful for definitively diagnosing disease or for eliminating breeders. It is not predictive of the development of disease. The SOD 1 seems to be near the locus for the DM gene, which is why it is associated with it in some cases.

Clemmons then went on to say that this focus on a test which is not predictive is drawing attention away from actually finding the locus (or loci) truly responsible for causing DM. He would like to see more work toward improved diagnostics. He also noted that similar disease presentations are being labelled DM, and many have not been shown to have the same pathogenesis (cause and development of disease) as the disease in German Shepherd Dogs. They may not have the same genetic pattern of inheritance at all.

It is possible that your girl does indeed have DM, but I would not use a positive SOD 1 test as confirmation of the diagnosis. In confirmed cases of DM, Dr. Clemmons has had dramatic success with the protocol that is outlined on his website, involving exercise,

diet, supplements, and two medications, as well as supportive treatments.

I am concerned that your dog may have another spinal cord disease which looks somewhat like DM and that, in the presence of a positive SOD 1 test, your vet may have diagnosed DM. Many older dogs develop mild proprioceptive deficits, which means that they don't always know where their hind feet are, and they may drag their toes at times. This is not the same as DM; it is usually much less serious. Dogs can also develop disc problems which can mimic DM. Disc diseases are treated differently from DM. I urge you to work with a vet who is willing to pursue a more definitive diagnosis, if that is what you want. It is hard to give advice about therapeutic options when we are not certain of the problem.

I will say that I have had good success treating dogs with both proprioceptive problems and disc disease. I have used constitutional homeopathic prescribing and acupuncture. You might consider looking for a vet in your area who offers these services, if it turns out the DM was diagnosed on the basis of the flawed SOD 1 genetic test.

Regards,

Sara

S.F. Chapman DVM, MRCVS, VetMFHom

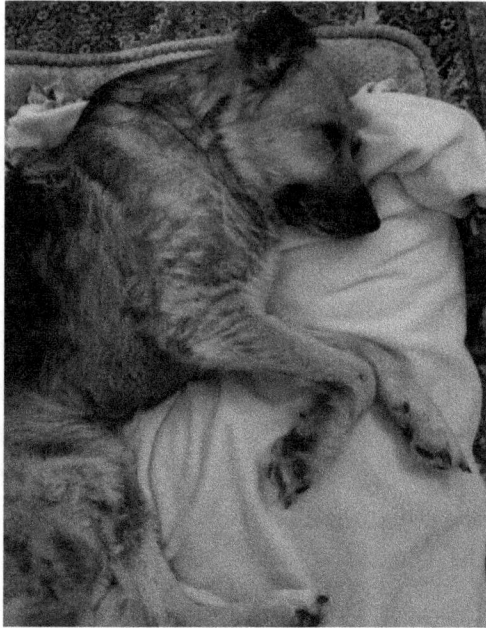

After the Spa

April 8

I HAD A WONDERFUL DAY! I went to the "spa" and got heat put on my hips, had electro therapy, acupuncture physical therapy (had to stand on this round thing that wobbled and practice putting weight on my hind legs) and I had hydrotherapy! I am one relaxed girl and my mom and dad can even tell my muscles are relaxed by the feel of my shoulders and my back. And, I used all four legs in the hydrotherapy tub! Dr. Ruth West was just wonderful with me and even got in the tub with me to show me what she wanted me to do. I went sound to sleep at the "spa" and snored!

I can't even tell you how much it means to me and to my family that I am getting some relief from sore shoulders and very weary front legs. I'm so fortunate to be able to do this thanks to your love, encouragement and support. Dr. Ruth West talked with us a long time and gave us things to do at home too! There are a lot of things that help without this extensive "spa" stuff so we will increase my daily massages and my mom and dad will be positioning me to stand on all fours when I stand up. I can have a heating pad on my hips if I like it; I'm getting joint nutrition and essential oils all with really good food. We will be putting my front feet up on a stool to help me remember to use my back legs and shift my weight. We couldn't have done all this without our Ginger Harness but now need to move to a Help Em Up Harness so my mom can manage me without help. It's ordered and should be here Tuesday. It's a happy day at our house.

Dear God, please bless the beasts and the children.

April 9, 2016

Today was restful and I was able to get up on my own the whole day whenever I wanted to. There is something I am excited to show you but we all have to wait a few days so I can share the photos with you! I had a professional photo shoot!!!!! More to follow about that!

My mom and dad are feeling that therapy was a good thing and I think so too. They are all about whatever is going to make me comfortable. My therapy doc is 35 minutes from home and we will be going twice weekly for as long as I am able and as long as we see good things from it. This is a gift from all of you who have prayed for me and who pray daily for the abused, neglected and homeless pets. Prayers do work. Healing positive energy works. .... Maybe not always the way we pray for, but always the way of the universe, the way of goodness in the long run. Be strong and of good faith.

How we got lucky enough to find Dr. Ruth West at a veterinary practice in Raleigh, I'll never know. Her concentration is physical therapy and pain management for dogs, and we have hit the jackpot. I knew I was in the right place the moment I walked in. The calm

103

loving atmosphere went right to my heart. Oh, that every dog in pain could be blessed enough to have this treatment.

April 11, 2016

All is well here! I got to go out in the yard and lie on my blanket today in the warm sun. I didn't stay long but enough time to nose around the blooming snowball bush and stick my nose in the planter. I was up most of the day without a nap so I am weary tonight and my folks can tell because I don't want to move. I'm on my "your bed " with my water bowl right next to me. I have my boots on because my mom thinks I may need to go out in the middle of the night. I am getting really delicious meals and it's hard to believe I weigh 75 pounds now. My dad and mom are being cautious about how much I eat and what I eat to make sure my body doesn't get too heavy for my wobbly legs. DM is such a cruel disease because my mind is perfect!

If my mind and my hind could just get together!

April 12, 2016

It was my second therapy day and I'm pretty tired but happy. I had a full day again of acupuncture and hydro and physical therapy. I am so blessed! It's hard to believe a one-time throw away dog like me is now blessed enough to be saved, to be warm and fed, to have your bed(s), to have a mom and dad, to have a home, to be getting therapy. All of you good people restore my parents' faith in humanity. I have a new harness called a "Help Em Up " and it helps my mom and dad get me in and out of the house and car. Mom will send pics tomorrow.

April 13, 2016

Well, I got my mom up at 3:00 am and at 6:30 am and I've been awake ever since. I'm not very mobile today but needed a day of lying around after therapy yesterday. My mom spent the morning figuring out that it's hard to put on my new harness with me lying down. I didn't know what to think about that thing but she finally got it on right. I had to go outside so badly by the time she figured it out that I didn't care how it felt. I'm very aware of every move that goes on around me and not at all happy when I want something and figure my dad or mom should know why I'm whining. Annie has come to lie beside me because she knows I'm fretting over something. I still love catching the ball even if I can't go after it. My mom has gotten pretty good about retrieving...

Once again my Facebook Family fills my heart with love and appreciation. My family is awed by your spirits and your support.

April 15, 2016

Sorry I didn't post yesterday. It wasn't a good day anyway and today I am in therapy all day. Will send post later but I am in good hands! I got the nicest gift box today from my special friends, Rex, Juni, Baby Girl, Simba, Albi, Mr. B, Kitty, Peterman, Zebo, And Eddie. They sent me such nice cards and they follow me every single day. It was wonderful to come home from a day of therapy to the nice presents. I had a good day at therapy too! I walked on my own afterward to go outside and my doctor was really happy with what I was able to do.

So many of you have sent us the most unimaginable gifts to help Sandy. Without these gifts and the donations you have so generously given to her GoFundMe account, we could never afford to sustain her and provide her with the comforts she has. She does not lack for anything. She has so many who love her and yet she is one in thousands of dogs who are suffering from DM. Sandy is one lucky girl to have the love of all of you.

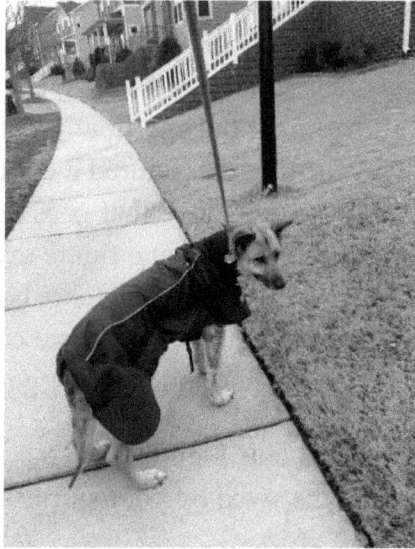

April 16, 2016

I had a decent day and this afternoon I was up on my own three times. I wanted to play with Annie and nosed her several times but she's an old stick in the mud and wouldn't cooperate. My harness has been a big help to my mom and dad to get me to the yard. I've learned that whining gets their attention so I am doing it a lot. Tomorrow may be training on wheels day... depending on how I feel after breakfast!

The big old Cane Corso next door woofs at us like a big bad meanie but when I go to the fence he runs away... bahahahaha!

So here's a thought I had today while lying in the sunshine for a few minutes. If every one of my Facebook friends would also add "and bless all the homeless animals" to their prayer for me, then maybe the goodness will find its way to some of them.

Today was a little better! I got up on my own three times and got to lie outside and enjoy some sunshine for a few minutes. The harness is a real help to mom and dad getting me to the yard and I don't mind it at all. I felt good enough to ask Annie to play but she was pretty stuck up about it so my mom threw the ball to me. Therapy seems to help my back be straighter and relaxes the muscles in my shoulders. My mom says it may be training wheels day tomorrow depending on how I feel.

So, I was thinking today when I was outside that if every single one of my Facebook friends was to add a little tiny prayer for all the homeless and neglected animals, then surely some good would come of it.

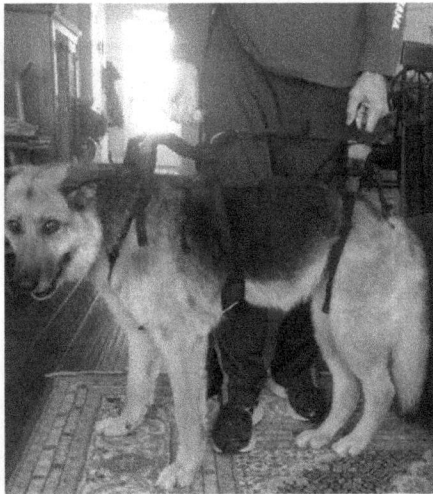

April 17, 2016

It was an exhausting day and all of us are worn out! I spent time in my wheels today! I did so well, and even though it was stressful, I soon tried my best to get down the walkway to the back door with my wheels on. Not a good move!

My mom is making me lie on my left side because the fur on my right side is wearing off from lying down on it so much. I'm a real sight with the wheel harnesses over my HEU harness. We will try to take pictures tomorrow. I did figure out how to move around the yard and maybe I'll actually like it if I use it some more. Tomorrow...and tomorrow will be another day for one more of us to be saved.

She scared me to death today. Our back porch is elevated by two steps and it is brick. She tried to get over the steps while still in her wheels, and it was one of those slow-motion moments. I couldn't get to her fast enough, and then she was all tangled in the wheels. All of us were a bit traumatized, but we went in and just calmed down. Man, is she hard-headed!

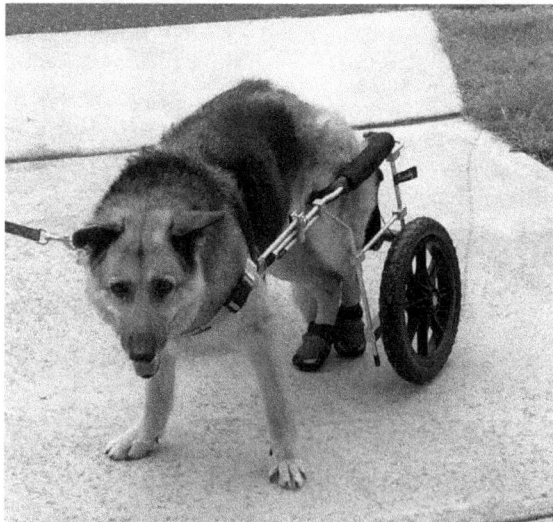

April 19, 2016

Tired.... I had therapy today and did well. My back legs are still trying to work and occasionally I get up on them by myself. I'm not a happy camper tonight because my mom is making me sleep on my left side.

I'm getting bedsores on my right side because that's the side I lay on all the time. It seems my doctor told my mom to try to put me on my left side. When she does it I wait until she walks away and then I work my way over back to my right side, hoping she won't notice. However, I'm on my bed ready for sleep and it looks like mom won. I don't have the energy I had earlier today so I can't fight her. She didn't realize how strong I am when I don't want to do something.

Wheels again tomorrow. It is beginning to look like I'm going to need them most of the time from now on until the DM starts to take the use of my front legs. We are all thankful today was good.

April 20, 2016

You won't believe this. We had a not so good few minutes in my wheels again when I took off for the steps. When I couldn't go up I reared up and flipped over before my mom could get to me. Guess I didn't learn my lesson the first time. I wasn't hurt, a bit scared, but I recovered nicely by the afternoon. And just to show my parents that I don't need those wheels yet, I walked around the yard, went to the fence three times, and laid in the yard all on my own. I got to act like a dog all afternoon and my mom even put a bed out on the sidewalk for me. It was glorious! A reminder: a breath of air and warm sunshine is a wonderful blessing. I hope each one of you had a good day.

April 21, 2016

I went outside today and held myself up for a few steps. It broke my heart to fall at the end but I was proud anyway. Still a big accomplishment for two days in a row although today was not as good as yesterday.

Back to therapy tomorrow.

April 22, 2016

Another very long day of therapy and multiple "accidents" in car and house. We are all worn out. My protein is too high and mom went all over looking for a good food for me. I will NOT eat fish...and I turned my nose up at beef rice and sweet potatoes. I also have the beginnings of a UTI so am on Clavamox. Will only do one day of therapy next week. I need a low-protein grain-free diet. None to be found. Will look for more tomorrow.

Lesson of the day: Sandy will NOT eat fish, and when she decides she isn't going to eat, she means it. I won't repeat that trial again. Multiple tries yielded nothing but food all over the floor and a stubborn Sandy. She even tried turning her head in the opposite direction of the spoon. Reminded me of my child when I first offered her carrots. They ended up in my face, on my shirt, and in my hair. And not at all in her mouth.

April 23, 2016

I got some much-needed rest today. I am now sleeping on a donut for relief on my almost a bedsore spot. I was picky at breakfast but ate that boiled chicken and rice so fast it felt amazing!! I'm taking some kind of cranberry treats and started my antibiotic for my UTI. I got up on my own several times enough to go from one side of the couch to my bed. Mom cooked enough chicken breast and rice for all day tomorrow and Monday. At this rate we will need to buy chicken every other day....my folks will go to the pet store that carries a lot of specialty stuff tomorrow.

Just so people understand..... My mom and dad are not trying to be heroes by saving me or keeping me alive. They know that when the light is no longer in my eyes and I am not having a good time, it will be time for me to travel on across the Rainbow Bridge to my next forever home. They know that there are so many of you that deal with sick and disabled fur babies and they thank each one of you for loving God's creatures through all the sacrifice. They only hope to be a small voice for all of them and to help understand that we have the power to save them all by increasing awareness and compassion. They don't feel like they deserve any more credit than anyone in this position but they do feel a responsibility to inform, to set an example, and to recognize that we are all in this together.

Love and peaceful rest to all.

It has been on my mind a lot about how to pay back all the kindnesses that have been extended to Sandy. I've come to the decision that the best thing we can do is to pay it forward. So, I will continue to be Sandy's voice and journal her successes and failures, her journey. Perhaps one day I'll write a book. The connection on social media with people from all over the world who are reading about Sandy's story is overwhelming. Who ever knew that a neglected, mange-covered German Shepherd could touch so many people?

April 24, 2016

I thought this comment from my namesake would be precious to all of you. She is the one who was determined that I be rescued. Without her I would not be here:

From Sandy's saving grace, Sandra:

"Sandy was such a special girl at the shelter. As horrible as she looked and as sick as she was, she wanted to live - it was so obvious in her struggle to stand and the sparkle in her eyes. Out of all the less fortunate dogs I have worked with, Sandy was on top of the list for a miracle. She got her miracle. Every dime that has been spent on her to make her healthy, every ounce of energy that's used to keep her

going, is not a waste. She wanted to live and will let you know when she's ready to go."

April 25, 2016

I had a busy day. Well, busy for me anyway. After breakfast I moved around a bit more than the past few days. Then this afternoon I walked around the yard and did the dog thing: checked out the fence, sniffed all the mulch, and enjoyed the view from the patio on my "your bed". And, of course, I made sure I covered up the spots where Buddy and Annie had made a smell!

Thanks to so many of my friends and family, my mom ordered Eddie's Wheels for me today!!!! The other wheels were just not working for my size, and the metal bracket to the backstops broke off of both sides when I flipped them over. We got the story about the first wheels I had from the owner of EDDIE'S WHEELS and it seems the man who owns that business sends all the manufacturing to China and blatantly misleads people who look for durable quality wheels. Hope you haven't had problems with yours if you own them. Anyway, it will be a little over two weeks before my EDDIE'S WHEELS get here and maybe then I can really take walks with my family again.

We sincerely thank you for all the supportive comments and notes to us after receiving a less-than-gracious comment on Sandy's page. We know that all of you are with us in your hearts as we are with each of you in your journey here with all of God's creatures.

Diana and Michael (mom and dad).

April 26, 2016

Well, I must say that I know I never have to worry about you all having my back or my parents' backs! You are all amazing! Wouldn't it be cool to have an animal lovers' convention! We are such an amazing force when on a mission!

I had a quiet day today. Mom was working and dad was out off and on. So I am demanding a lot of attention this evening! It even paid off with a bone!

Started my B12 and I'm waiting to see if the ability to walk a bit continues. The counter on the side of the kitchen looks like a vitamin and supplement store however those cranberry chews work wonders!! Mom broke open vitamin E capsules and put it on the raw spots on my hind legs and they are so much better. I had licked them raw because of the UTI and now feel better! Maybe I'll make a list and post it of all the supplements I take in case it will help another ailing four-legged person.

Yes, one of our kitchen counters looks like a chemistry lab or a pharmacy counter. I feel so lucky to have discovered some supplements and vitamins that help her. She seems so grateful for any kindness offered to her, except fish.

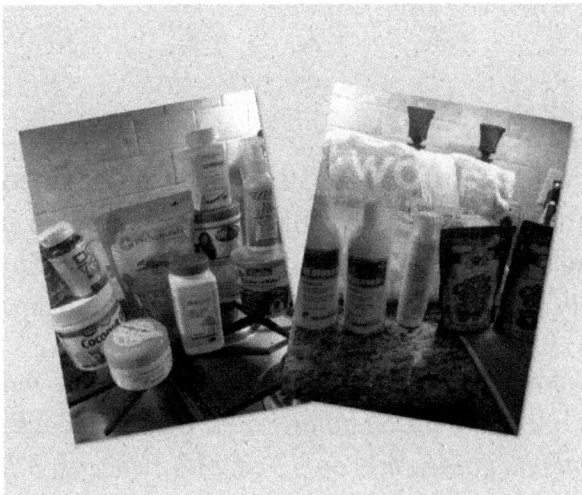

April 27, 2016

It was therapy day today and Dr. Ruth was pleased that I did well. I am very tired tonight but went out in the yard and walked around a bit earlier.

I am living proof that the healing energy created through prayer and constant love does work! Even if it works for a day here and there!!!! I love the fresh smells like grass, and the coleus on the patio, the way the birds gather on the fence waiting their chance at the feeder, the smell of chicken on the grill, the thrill of standing on my own, simple things that are life's blessings I never had before. Now for a night of wonderful deep sleep!

For many years, I have tried the practice of being grateful and looking at the glass as half full. It has helped so many times in stressful situations and in times of wanting to feel sorry for myself. The poor dogs in this world who never know the comfort of a bed, of safety, of food, of love... it is such a huge problem in our world, and there is so much to do to save them all. However, every little effort counts, every penny counts, every kind thought and every prayer offered makes it all worth it when you save just one!

April 28 2016

My posts will be off a little this weekend. I'm home with dad weathering the storms with Annie and Buddy. Mom is off with my auntie doing sister things. My dad is awesome for taking care of all of us especially when it requires hiding in the closet from the thunder!

The mental picture of my 6'5" husband in the master bedroom closet with one German Shepherd on a bed, one cocker spaniel mix on a bed and one golden mix on a bed, plus two cats, all of our clothes and shoes, is quite humorous. Bless his heart for gathering all the household members to keep them safe. The storm passed (not soon enough for the temporary residents of the closet), and all are ok.

April 30, 2016

I'll be back with daily highlights and lowlights tomorrow. Dad has been great and I am glad he is so good about remembering my pills and my mom is having a nice time. I'd like each of my friends to say special prayers tonight for the lost fur babies. There was one in my neighborhood today.

May 2, 2016

So here I am on a Monday evening after the hail and thunder. I had a good weekend with my dad and was glad to see my mom when she got home. I started some new food today; my mom is mixing organic freeze-dried veggies in with my food and so far it's pretty yummy.

Here's the list of my supplements and meds:

Rimadyl

Tramadol

Gabapentin

Cranberry Relief by Nature Vet

Omega 3 Chews

EFAC for Joint Health

Dasaquin

DGP By American Bio Sciences

Methyl B12

Senior-Vite by Nutri-Vet

Coconut Oil

And that takes up one whole part of the counter!

May 3, 2016

My new diet to lower the protein in my blood includes an amazing cup of freeze-dried vegetables that smell so good my mom thought about fixing them for dinner. I love the food...At least I mean I loved it the past three meals.

My wheels can't get here soon enough. I am one determined girl and I want to play so badly, but my back legs just won't work enough to rely on them. The good news is that so far my front legs are working fine. I've been very active but fussy today, because I am frustrated that I can't play with Annie without falling and I want attention so much! I went my whole life without ear rubs and back scratches so now I can't get enough of them. And today I was very insistent about NOT lying on my left side. My folks say my strong will is what helped me survive the abuse and neglect.

So, tomorrow is therapy day, and I've had pretty good days since my last session so maybe it will continue to help me.

Thank you all my loyal friends and I hope all of you know you mean a lot to me. Remember that Mother's Day is another day to honor your favorite mom with a donation of any size to a rescue organization!

Veterinary medicine has come so far! We are so blessed to have veterinary advice and care by veterinarians who treasure the life of each dog!

May 5, 2016

It's been a soggy day, and I'm not so full of pep when it is rainy and damp. I was full of energy last night at bedtime and insisted on sleeping on my right side. My mom finally gave up. Today Bella, Bucket and Peter came to stay for a long weekend. So here are six dogs and two cats and two humans who have to clear hurdles every time they move. Dad thinks we are a zoo and meal time around here is a major production..... Thus, mom and dad ate tuna sandwiches tonight. It is still thundering and we don't like the lightning and there are too many of us for the closet.

This degenerative myelopathy stuff is just happening to too many dogs. It's so heartbreaking to know that so many of us will end up not being able to use our legs, so tonight I'd like to ask each of you to pray for a veterinarian who does therapy, who researches to find the cure, who lovingly explains to humans what this disease means, and pray for the future veterinarians who are studying so hard and will incur tremendous debt in order to be our doctors and specialists.

May 6, 2016

Ok.... so, I wrote a whole post tonight and somehow deleted it so here it is in abbreviated form:

I played with Peter today while mom held me up in my harness.

It has rained for five days and I'm ready for sunshine.

117

I haven't had Tramadol in 4 days but have been whining tonight so mom will get Tramadol tomorrow. I was very active and engaged without it but my folks are worried that I might be uncomfortable; I still have the UTI situation and am still on antibiotics.

A puppy mill in Virginia was raided today and many dogs saved. Kudos to the rescuers and fosters!

May 9, 2016

It was a very busy Mother's Day here with me, Buddy, Annie, Bucket, Bella, Peter, Tipper and Lulu, Rachael and Freddy and Anita and Kevin. We all had a beautiful day and lots of good food. Mom felt badly that we didn't get the good burgers and hot dogs so she got us elk horns! We were all pooped so we didn't post last night.

My parents have put me back on Tramadol twice a day because I seemed a little uncomfortable on my left side. I'm on a very expensive diet so they make sure I'm not getting grains and too much protein. My food runs about $68 a week, not nearly as cost-effective as Annie's and Buddy's.

But it has a lot of the nutrients that we believe are holding off the rapid advancement of my spinal issues. I am a bit stubborn about the left side thing but I am still good about waiting to use the bathroom outside.

You know, I'm thinking the older dogs in the shelters are there because people don't want to have to deal with their health issues. It's so so sad that they are there and don't understand why their person left them. It breaks my heart. My mom says some people are put on earth to care for people and some people are put here to take care of animals. She says she couldn't take care of a person like she does me. I'm thankful for all of you who are caring for your aging and diseased pets. You make a big difference in this world.

I don't think I will ever understand how people just forsake an animal if they have to move or if the animal gets sick, or how someone tosses an animal out of a car or other horrendous things we all know about. I hope every person reading this is part of the effort to make abusing and neglecting dogs a felony. As I write this, this kind of behavior is overlooked in too many states. If man is given dominion over all creation, how can we overlook our responsibility to take care of these voiceless creatures. As I have grown both in age and wisdom, I do understand that I am less if I am not caring for animals.

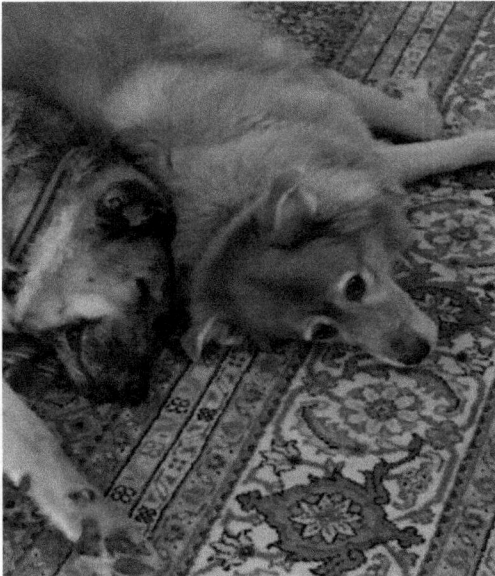

Sandy and Annie

<u>May 11, 2016</u>

Mom had to laugh at the post she wrote last night. She was half asleep when she wrote it and being the grammar nerd that she is, she was a bit horrified at all the misspelled words and things that were not even words! So she edited the post and corrected the misspelling.

I had therapy today and it seems I have now developed a skin problem where the HEU (Help Em UP) harness rubs my tummy so now we have even MORE medicine. And, to top it off I am having to sleep with a bolster between my hind legs to let air circulate to help clear up the problem. Dad had an appointment this morning so didn't go with mom to take me, then mom went to work and picked me up right after. Three times of lifting me all by herself was not her favorite task of the day.

I had an OK day at therapy (love that acupuncture and slept through it) but we avoided the hydrotherapy today because of the skin thing.

So many things happen to us when we get a spinal condition or lose the use of legs. We have to be watched for urinary tract infections, bedsores, skin scalding from urine, proper diet to avoid constipation, sore places where we scrape our feet, and skin irritations...... But, I am one happy girl to have my comfy "your beds" and my Annie and Buddy and my HOME! I know there are so many of us who don't have the good life I do, so tonight I hope one day there will be no homeless pets.

You have all been so loyal and kind to Sandy and to us as we journey through this debilitative disease with her. There are so many moments when I wish I could record her or capture a picture just to share it. Sometimes she can be quite the drama queen, and other days, tough as nails. She can be silly and moans when she wants something that isn't in reach. She barks when a strange dog is outside of our fence, and she snores in concert with her dad. She is a true survivor, and we have very high hopes her new wheels will help all of us include her in many walks and hikes. Our lives and our appreciation for dogs with these kinds of disabilities have been enriched by caring so deeply for her

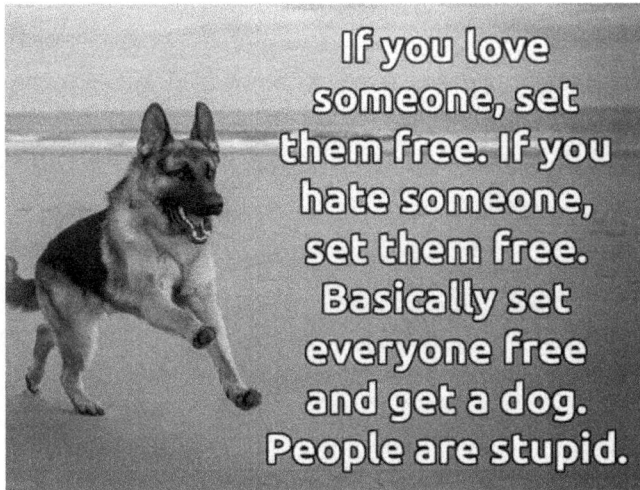

May 12, 2016

A walk!!!! I went on my wheels for a walk! The terrain around here is many hills and not many flat places but I went from behind the house in the alley to the end of the block (3 houses down) and back up the front. It was exciting to be out in the yard and there were so many things to sniff! I don't mind the bolster between my legs when I am lying down so my rash is improving.

Good news today. A friend of ours, a veterinarian in Florida, adopted a dog who had no home and it made us very happy!

My mom says if she was just beginning a career she would buy a lot of land and create a place like **Best Friends Animal Sanctuary** (www.bestfriends.org) in Utah. She says it is the most wonderful place she's ever been and she's been to the Vatican (with a private audience with the pope) and she's been to the Eiffel Tower, and Normandy and beaches everywhere and dad has been to Italy and Israel and all over Europe..... but they say if they didn't have family here they'd move to Kanab, Utah to volunteer at **Best Friends Animal Sanctuary (www.bestfriends.org)** every day.

A few years ago, one of my lifelong friends, Dr. Joan DaVanzo, and I journeyed to Best Friends in Kanab, Utah, to volunteer. I had become aware of the mission and rescue work of Best Friends when they rescued over 20 of the abused pit bulls from Virginia's most well-known dog abuser, Michael Vick. It was a life-changing experience and reached into my soul. The animal sanctuary is built on sacred Indian spiritual ground, and with every whisper of the desert wind and in the face of every animal there, you know that you are experiencing a holy and sacred space. The people there are fulfilled in ways many of us only hope to be, and live in the spirit of giving. I was blessed with this experience and carry it in my heart every day.

May 13, 2016

Another day, another walk. And on this day I left unwelcome presents for my mom on the den rug. I needed to go out and wasn't able to wake mom or dad....... so.......

But mom got it all taken care of and we went on a walk this afternoon. About 100 meters. I liked it a lot and the hill was a challenge but I did it.

This picture is of Lulu. She is not allowed outside, but right after the thunderstorm last night she ran out the back door when mom was taking me out. Mom tried to catch her but the little stinker ran through the fence. Mom had to hold me up and couldn't run after her. About

30 minutes later she was howling at the back door. She's a bit whacko. She tries to climb the wall in the shower, she tries to jump on things and misses. Actually she can be quite entertaining but I think it's because she's not the brightest crayon in the box!

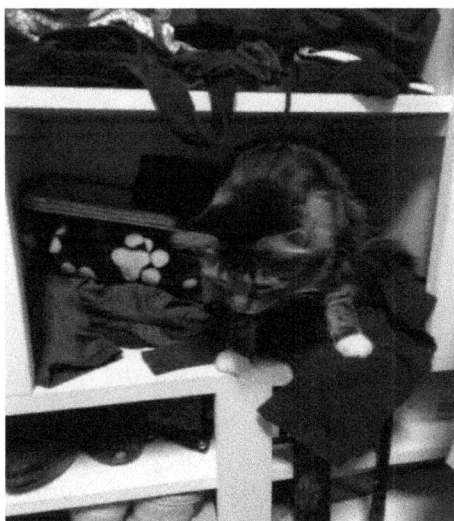

Lulu up to no good

May 14, 2016

By the time my mom got home it was looking like rain so we all went for a short walk. It was shorter than planned because it did start to rain. So now we are dried off and inside for a nice calm Saturday night. I didn't leave any presents this morning and it seems the more I walk with my wheels the more I'm willing to try to walk. I'm doing more dragging myself around than before when indoors and not in my wheels, and my dad and mom try not to think about what that means. My wheels are a blessing and I'm so grateful for the love that helps me every day. From my vitamins to my wheels, from my "your bed" to my harness, from my treats to my boots... it's all really amazing. I have one more therapy session and then we will decide what to continue.

My mom has a concert to perform tomorrow so don't worry if I don't post tomorrow!

May 15, 2016

Brief update tonight. I have terrible diarrhea and am not feeling too good. Looks like chicken and rice time. I didn't go on a walk today and I'm now to the point where I can only take about four steps without my hind legs failing. Good thing my dad has big muscles to take me out and pick me up. Mom is not too bad either.

Speaking of mom, she sings with the **North Carolina Master Chorale.**

We will find out this Wednesday if Dr. Ruth West thinks I should continue therapy with all the treatments or maybe have some laser treatments. Right now I'm just thankful for the comfy "your bed" and the safety of home and all the blessings you send me!

May 16 2016

I'm sorry I didn't post pictures of our walk today. I did better and walked a long way compared to before. But it is much more work now to get me outside and it has to be pretty immediate when I want to go because of my diarrhea. I'll go to the vet if not better tomorrow. It seems the spinal issues are progressing because now when I get my back legs crossed I can't get them unwound. I scoot around the den and don't have much use of my back end.

To all of you out there who are dealing with the harnesses and the wheels and the cleaning feet, legs, and tails, after every bathroom incident, you are in our thoughts and prayers. The constant washing of blankets, changing protective disposable pads, and being on duty 24/7 are your routine, as it is ours. God bless you for your love and patience, and may we all continue this journey with grace and compassion.

May 17, 2016

I have two comfortable "your beds" and tomorrow Mom and Dad will buy some inexpensive rugs at Walmart to put down over the carpet. I can't seem to make it outside to the bathroom and it's the best way to keep the good carpet clean. Your prayers and love are so appreciated and all of you have no idea how much strength you give me and mom and dad. Mom says that at the end of the day when her shoulders ache and Dad's back hurts, your encouragement is like a breath of fresh air and it helps her know she can do it again tomorrow.

To our wonderful Facebook family and friends:

Well, we don't feel like heroes much today, and really, we don't want to be. We get discouraged like many of you with ailing pets, and we aren't anything special because we chose to love and help this wonderful dog. We ask God to help us serve this creature, as she is one of His own, and we just take one day at a time. Thank you for all your messages and prayers and all the love. It makes a huge difference, not only to us but to all the people viewing this Facebook page and sharing this journey.

May 18, 2016

We needed every word you sent to me last night and prayers work again! Turns out I do have a bacterial imbalance in my intestines and I'm now on more meds. But I walked, well, tottered on my own four feet a bit today and ate all my dinner. I even went to the toy box and dragged out an old bone. I slept most of the night on my left side. Dad and mom kept me home from therapy because they were concerned I was under the weather. Turns out they were right.

Isn't it awe-inspiring how all your prayers and positive energies keep helping me. Think how many times you have made me better. Truly blessed.

When I think of prayers, I think of all the positive energies that are created. I think of the miracles that have resulted from prayers. I know that the prayers you send have such power over what is happening to Sandy and to us. It is humbling and so appreciated.

<u>May 20, 2016</u>

Have had a very busy couple of days. Well, not me really but my mom. I am feeling sooo much better and back to eating normally and able to get around a little bit on my own. We are hoping my regression was due to the bacterial infection in my digestive tract. How I got some bacteria no one knows. But my meds are helping and I am almost ready to try to catch the ball again provided I am lying down and the pitcher is accurate with the throw.

*Saw a post tonight on the Facebook page for **Trio Animal Foundation** that just made us speechless and heartbroken. Some poor fur baby had been found that was so matted, you couldn't even tell it was a dog. Why? Why? Why are some people so cruel? All of us on Facebook need to share the posts and bring these abusers to justice. Trio Animal Foundation is a very special rescue that saves the worst of the worst. You can follow them on Facebook.*

May 22, 2016

Well we had quite the adventure this past weekend and now that it is Sunday, we can share. My folks went out of town overnight. They have always used **PetnNanny** to care for Annie and Buddy and Tipper and Lulu, but had never left me with the others to be cared for by the pet sitter. Well, my pet sitter, Shannon, was so wonderful and I did absolutely great! I ate, I didn't mess in the house and it was all so much easier than my folks worried about! I was glad to see them when they got home but had no anxiety or intestinal problems so they were very happy. I'm wobbling around but not dragging as much as when I was sick. We think this is good. Thank you Shannon of **PetnNanny**!!!

We know so many of you give up trips and weekend excursions or visits because you don't have a good pet sitter. How we lucked out to find PetnNanny was another "gift". Leaving a disabled pet is so hard, so I want to thank Shannon and her people for giving me peace of mind.

May 23, 2016

My intestinal infection has calmed down a lot and that chicken and rice works wonders. I was so tired yesterday but got a bath anyway which I needed. I'm a bit perkier today.

Mom and Dad tried a standing bowl for me but since my back legs won't allow me to stand for long it doesn't work too well for me. I didn't really know how to eat out of a bowl when I first got here, and so I licked everything into the edges. Then mom or dad would stir it but it ended up more on the floor than in my tummy. Thus, the fork. I eat every forkful when I'm feeling good. My nose is long so my Dad feeds me with a fork. Actually, I rather like being fed with a fork instead of having to stick my beautiful nose down into the dish.

Hopefully it won't be rainy tomorrow and I can go for a walk.

Please pray for Trio Animal Foundation's most recent rescue who was so neglected his coat had formed a matted cocoon around him and his skin is rotting. Pray that one day in this world people won't hurt us anymore.

I have come to believe that people who hurt animals and neglect and abuse them are those whose souls are black. They are less evolved and unconscious about the dominion of the human race and its responsibilities.

May 24, 2016

Went on a walk today and it completely wore me out. I go to therapy tomorrow so my day has been calm except for a walk. I just hate lying on my left side and Mom and Dad are working hard to keep the spot on my hip bone from breaking open. Mom says she needs to be 35 again to do all the hauling and lifting; dad is very strong but has to be careful about his lower back (old football injury). I can still move my back legs but I don't have much feeling in them.

Mom joined the Degenerative Myelopathy group on Twitter. She doesn't know much about tweeting, but thinks it may be another way to increase awareness. Wish the American Kennel Club would recognize this terrible disease as a cause....

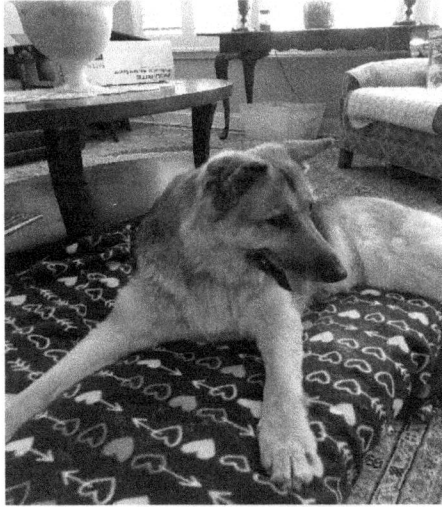

I'm a perky girl today

May 25, 2016

I didn't walk at all yesterday or this morning but I DID tonight! Celebrating walking across the den instead of dragging my hind legs! This disease is such a roller coaster and we are all thankful I can still control my bathroom needs because that is terrible when it happens. My mom and dad both say that if they ever become incontinent and have uncontrollable bowels they want to go to the journey beyond the rainbow bridge.

Our prayers go out to all you parents of four-legged children who have disabilities.... You are the inspiration, you are the hope, you are the embodiment of love. May you sleep well and wake to a joyful morning.

May 26, 2016

I had a really good day. I went to therapy today and they were so pleased with what I did. I have gotten around all day on all 4 legs with only a little help. We are all learning to live in the moment of joy and accomplishment. Each time I am able to stand or walk is a celebration and every moment I feel good a reason to be thankful. What a lesson ... Life is only moment to moment. None of us are promised the next minute or day or month or year. To live in each moment with all that we are and all that we have to give...that is the gift.

Sandy teaches us lessons every day. She shows undying loyalty, she tries with all of her strength, she never has a grouchy moment, she is gentle and appreciative. She has a pure trust that is so unbelievable, considering her abuse and neglect. When we are tired, her determination gives us strength. When we are frustrated, she is calm. When we are less than, she is more.

May 28, 2016

I want to remember and thank and honor all military service dogs who serve this country and those who gave their lives so we can be free.

If you are not aware that some service dogs return home to only have no home, please research them. So many need special homes and loads of love. They gave for our country, and we surely owe them. Check out:

http://www.servicedogs.org
https://freedomservicedogs.org
https://www.thesprucepets.com
https://servicedogsva.org

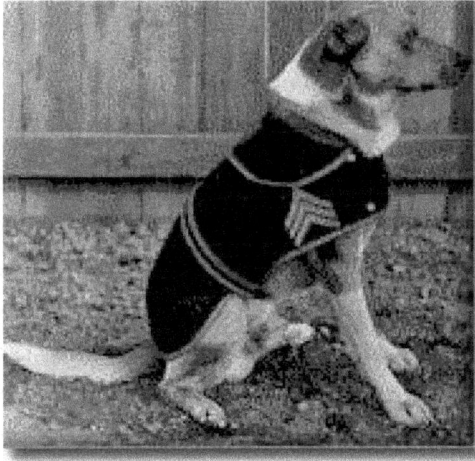

<u>May 29, 2016</u>

I had a nice walk last night and I'm still doing my best to get around. I am very determined and wake my dad up every morning very early because that's when I need to go out.

My mom and dad went to a Memorial Day barbecue today. Mom's dad landed at Normandy in WW II and served under General Patton. Dad's father was in the Navy. It's so sad that the younger generation has such a small understanding of what their grandparents fought and died for and that they could even believe a word from a socialist politician. Their grandparents died for their freedom and for our constitution and rights. So much they don't comprehend about how a man like Hitler can socialize a whole nation and send thousands and thousands who disagreed with him to the gas chambers.

Oh my. I didn't mean to get all political but my mom's dad got her the very first kitty and dog she ever had and he loved animals so much. She owes a lot to him for teaching her about animals and how to love them.

Say a prayer for our two and four-legged troops in harm's way tonight and tomorrow and always.

My dad brought me my first kitten when I was two years old. I named her DeeDee (most likely because I could not say "kitty"). From then on, we always had cats. I got my first dog when I was seven. She was an English Cocker, and I named her Tammy. She lived until I was 16, and when she died, I cried for days. I have gone on to have two more cockers, Happy and Sunshine, then rescued a collie mix named Simone. Annie came into our lives when my daughter found her in the equestrian barn at her college in the wee hours of the morning. She was a six-week-old puppy someone had apparently just "dropped off". Then my girlfriend and I adopted Buddy from Best Friends, and now Sandy. I cannot imagine my life without a dog, and have come to realize that we save them one rescue at a time.

May 30, 2016

I had a nice walk today on my wheels in between thunder storms. Several neighbors stopped and wondered why I was on wheels and my mom got to share information about DM. So much research is needed and so much stem cell advancement needed and it seems soooooo slow to be available. So many of us have DM and so little is known about it.

We met a neighbor today who adopted a brother and sister from a rescue. We believe that once you rescue, you'll never ever pay for a purebred high-dollar designer dog again. You can find plenty of them in rescue organizations.......

My meds are stable and I'm still able to get up and walk to get water. I get antsy in the evening if I have had a walk so we will try every day, weather permitting.

Prayers tonight for all the pitiful dogs being held in puppy mills and who never know a gentle touch or a blade of grass. Those who are caged and cannot even stand up to walk around...May angels ease their pain.

If I ruled the world, it would be criminal with severe penalties for hurting an animal. There are many areas of the USA where puppy mills breed dogs in the filthiest, most horrible conditions. Pennsylvania Amish and southwest Virginia are awful. Rural law enforcement often looks the other way when a resident is participating in puppy mill activity and is not providing proper shelter or food to animals. Breeders are often at fault for breeding a dog with a gene mutation that will be passed on to puppies. That is the case with DM. Breeders should be required by law to breed responsibly and provide genetic information to anyone who adopts.

June 1, 2016

It was sort of an uneventful day which gave me time to think about this DM thing. My mom read on the DM Facebook page that someone has written to Ellen DeGeneres to ask her to champion more dedicated research in the field of DM. I was thinking that if every single one of my Facebook friends would email Ellen's show or tweet it on a lot of pages, maybe we could help make this happen. So, my mom is going to try it and we all hope you will too! We are a voice of thousands of fur babies who suffer from this and no one is truly speaking out. There is no specific treatment and no specific cure and even the diagnosis is sketchy. Veterinarians come out of vet school usually in debt for college loans and veterinary charges in practices are more than what they would be for humans. This seems so backwards to me and so we will try our hashtags and our tweets and our FB page to raise hearts and minds towards help for this disease. I know you; my faithful and living friends will help too!

June 3, 2016

Ok, so my mom has gone for the weekend and it's us and Dad! My mom is spending a long weekend with Rachael (my human sister) in NYC, so Dad is on full-time duty. I got up at 2 and went out and Mom got dressed and now I'm confused because we had to go back to bed...What time is it anyway?

June 4, 2016

My mom is home, I ate all 4 cups of food and I'm stretched out in my usual spot! Mom got delayed coming home and was in the airport for many many hours and got no sleep last night so she napped today. Dad was so good while she was gone and he got up early every morning, took me out in the middle of the night, and couldn't have been better. I guess we are all creatures of habit and all of us are feeling cozy and comfy with the whole family at home. Mom says she notices that I am dragging myself around more, so two things are going to happen tomorrow. 1) I'll be out on my wheels and 2) my bed in my playpen will be where I stay when they go out. Mom says I can't afford the bedsore breaking open.

I've finished my rounds of physical therapy and now we have to make the decision how to keep up the acupuncture and laser therapy. My doctor, Dr. Ruth West is leaving the veterinary practice and opening her own mobile practice to do acupuncture and laser therapy so she will be able to come to me. Which saves the two-hour trip each week but we have to figure out the cost of at-home visits.

On the news side, Tipper, who is an indoor cat, got very adventurous while mom was away and ran out of the front door when my dad opened it. He told her to get back in the house and she did, but her interest in the outdoors is not a good thing. She ran away one time in their old house for almost three months. She finally came home looking horrible and starving so Mom doesn't want her to go outside anymore. Seems she doesn't have the sense to come home if she gets out.

Thanks to all of you for missing my updates and for keeping me in your hearts!

June 8, 2016

It's birthday week at our house for both mom and dad. Annie and Buddy and I didn't even get a piece of cake! They said it would be bad for us because it was chocolate and even though we all tried our saddest eyes, they wouldn't give in.

I have a vet appointment at 10 in the morning due to blood in my stool.... Sorry for the graphic description but since I've shared most of my indignities with all of you before it seems like that's the only way to describe it. Mom took a sample in to vet today

I'm so glad to know that my Facebook family is learning from me and hope some dogs benefit from my experience. My mom swears the EFAC and Vitamin B12 (methyl) make a difference. And the Dasaquin too. Maybe one day stem cell treatment will be a routine healing practice and not so out of reach for dogs like me. I read the DM Facebook posts every day and my heart aches for my brothers and sisters suffering from this disease.

I do want to make sure each of you knows that prayers work! If your prayers hadn't worked, I would not be lying next to mom and dad's feet and I would have journeyed across that Rainbow Bridge months ago. Thanks to you I get to see the sunshine, I get to hear the thunder, I get to see the birds, lick my kitties, and eat the best meals I've ever had in my whole life. You also sustain my mom and dad and always help them to remember that the glass is half full!!

I am worried and nervous that we have to leave town for a funeral. We have a fabulous sitter, but taking care of Sandy is a lot to ask of someone. So, Rachael is going to stay here and pet sit. Thank goodness.

June 10, 2016

Mom and dad were away for a while at a funeral and Rachael was here with us.

Mom and dad are home now and I am worn out from taking a walk on my wheels. But it felt good to get outside and sniff around. Oh how I wish my legs would hold me up, and that there was some way to fix me. I have sparkling eyes and a gentle spirit; I am beautiful inside and out just like all my wonderful friends with DM. I am loyal and love attention...how did I get this way with my legs? Well, anyway, I will sleep well with my mom and dad home and maybe I will dream about running around with legs that work. Don't worry. I am ok!!!

Degenerative myelopathy is found in many breeds, but in particular in boxers and German Shepherds. Responsible breeders will have had the bloodlines checked to eliminate the possibility of DM. These genetic tests are expensive but the only way to ensure the dog will not pass DM to its offspring. It is a cruel disease, much like ALS (Lou Gehrigs Disease) and takes away the use of the body but leaves the brain intact, aware, cognizant, and incapable of communicating.

June 12

It's been a pretty good two days and the reason I didn't post last night is because my mom and dad celebrated their birthdays by going to see River Dance. They had a great time and it was pretty cool that I got to eat half of my dinner at 5:00 and the other half at 11:00. I've tried all

136

day today (with a little standing assistance from mom) to get Annie to play with me. I've head-butted her over and over and she's just too worried that I'd fall over to head butt me back. I was able to wobble on all 4 feet around the den today. I got a good ear cleaning and mom is going to set a vet appointment about my teeth because she thinks they may be bothering me. My teeth are in bad shape but I've been too weak to have them cleaned...I'm not fond of her putting her hand in my mouth so it's hard for her to see except she does see one that is broken.

Mom posted on the DM Facebook page today all the things she thinks have helped me supplement-wise and also the things that have helped me still be able to get around. My HelpEmUp harness has been a true lifesaver because dad is a former athlete and has a bad back and I am still stronger than my mom when I want to be.

Mom is calling Dr. Ruth tomorrow to schedule some acupuncture for me. We are going for a walk tomorrow evening in my wheels.

Sending our love to all of you and wishing you a night of peaceful rest.

Sometimes being tired is the only thing that keeps us from being discouraged. Too tired to think about it.

June 14, 2016

Who knows where these good days come from except from the prayers by all of you? I was full of myself today and played ball with mom, wobbled around the den all day and had some nice time in the yard to sniff and look and enjoy. We are all so blessed to have had this good day! I am so determined to stay strong and be a part of things! I am getting to enjoy simple things like rubs and hugs and just love my whole family. Thank you for the healing prayers and energies that you have sent my way!!!!

My mom is out of pocket tonight and Dad is on duty. There are many things that I love about my dad but most of all I love that he is so gentle and patient. He feeds me with a fork and gives me my meds with peanut butter. He's just the best!

There are so many holes in our world caused by hatred, abuse, intolerance, impatience, selfishness and greed. I am only one little speck in the universe but each of you has been loving and kind to me and for that I am grateful.

I am so blessed. Sandy's sweet dad is so willing to care for her and so good about seeing to her every need. Sandy is right. He is kindhearted and gentle and loves all of our four-legged children.

June 15, 2016

Mom is home! Dad had a big surprise last night! Annie is famous for counter surfing so when he went to the kitchen to refill his water, he took her with him. However, somehow his garlic Bologna and cheese sandwich made its way into my mouth and down to my tummy! He left it on the side table, so...

Mom had a good laugh at this. I walked to the door to greet her when she got home and this makes week two of being mobile enough to stand although wobbly and walk ok on carpet with only a few falters. See how much you are doing for me? Mom's motto is "Glass Half Full" and we are sending our love to all of you!

June 16, 2016

I was rubbing my mouth on the sides for a few days so my parents took me to vet....... YEAST! So I'm back to 2 to 3 baths a week with

Malaseb (mom will need chiropractor and massages) plus ear washes each time and eardrops. However, my mom put my no-slip socks on before we went to vet and I walked on their tile floor without falling! I'm still doing pretty well getting up and supporting myself with only a little help. Turns out my teeth are just worn and in pretty good shape considering. Wow! That was a surprise to mom and dad. So we will start the Malaseb tomorrow morning and here we go again.

Sandy looks like a deer when she walks with her socks on. She picks her feet up like there is something vile on them and puts one foot down at a time very carefully. It's hilarious, and she prances like a Tennessee Walker.

June 17, 2016

So it's the big glass box day tomorrow........ Mom has put it on the "to-do" list and it looks like all 3 of us will be getting baths. No bologna sandwiches today, but, I did manage to get Annie to head butt me twice and swing her hind end around to knock me over!

My mom was back at the vet today to have the plastic tips put on Lulu's claws. She fights Mom like a tiger when mom tries to cut her nails so the vet puts the tips on.

I am officially a whiner. If I can't get the other dogs to play, I whine. If I can't get the rubs I want, I whine, when I can't reach my ball I whine. Mom and Dad worried the past months when I would whine and now they've figured it out, which means I don't quite get the immediate reaction I used to get.

Tonight, I'd like to ask you to add the service dogs to your prayers. They are so smart and so much attuned to special needs, souls who hurt, and to our servicemen and women and our uniformed officers. They don't get near the recognition they deserve.

A few tips on the successful use of the big glass box:

Line the bottom with a heavy cotton bathmat and soak it before taking the dog into shower. Make sure to have a handheld attachment that reaches the bottom of the shower. Be prepared to be soaked, so don't wear anything but old clothes. Set dry towels just outside of the big glass box. For a GSD, you will need 4.

June 19, 2016

It's been bath and beauty weekend at our house. All three of us characters in the big glass box. Mom did an extra long one for me so I could soak in all the shampoo to help get rid of yeast on my skin. I pretty much loved the rubdown! Dad got a tee shirt from us that says "Best Dog Dad Ever" and he's worn it all day! After all the baths mom went out and finished planting stuff on the new walkway which I really like because it's not so far down. Dad had to spray the outside for bugs because mom found a nest of spiders. She hates spiders. Hope all the dog dads and foster dads had an especially nice day! I've been in my new home now for 5 full months and love being with my family!

More update tomorrow. It's been a busy day and we have a present for Dad in the morning and a card.

Will take pics and send them!!!

Happy Father's Day to all of my Facebook Dads who so lovingly take care of my canine and feline friends. My love to all of you!

June 20, 2016

I had a pretty laid back normal day. I'm not able to go outside by myself because I can't hold myself up to do either 1 or 2, so dad and mom always help me. Good news is I am still aware of needing to go out and haven't had any accidents in the house for some time. I get up by myself and wobble on all 4 feet to drink my water and only need help walking on the hardwood floors. Mom swears it is the Dasaquin and the Methyl B12 ..... But I'm also still getting the pain meds. I tried bumping Tipper several times today but she ignored me. I've been sleeping some nights on my left side without putting up a fuss. I get a rubdown most nights when I go to bed. Not bad, huh?

You know, I heard mom talking the other day and she mentioned that the states of North Carolina and South Carolina are still putting hundreds of dogs to sleep every day in shelters. If you know about any of them, your voice in a nice way can help change this and maybe one day there will be no more kill shelters. An email to your local SPCA or county shelter followed by an email to your state representative and senator does make a difference!

It is not as easy as it should be to send letters or emails to your state representatives. However, they really do make a difference, and if you type in your state plus .gov (www.va.gov is an example), you can usually find your representative's email. And always remember to call your local animal control/animal care facility to report suspected abuse, hoarding or improper housing for animals.

June 21, 2016

And, we went for a stroll today... on wheels of course...one block! I'm really pooped, but was able to sit and beg for part of mom's dinner. I whined until she got my ball from under the table and am now stretched out on the rug waiting for the last time outside before bedtime. My poor dad is getting up at 6 every morning to take me out since I've decided that's when I want to wake up.

I'm really doing as well as I've done since being totally down for a while and am going on over 3 weeks of being able to get around while on the rug. My ear drops are NOT my favorite thing. I have a spot on my right side that when mom scratches it my right hind leg does the scratching motion really well, so I think now it's part of my therapy. My "your bed" is all clean and smelling fresh, my water bowls are full and my heart if overflowing with gratitude for all of you, my Facebook Family.

June 22, 2016

I'm so glad I didn't run for office! The things people say about each other are just not good for the positive life I need so I can be healthy.

Anyway the good news is that we have baby blue birds hatched in our birdhouse, the frogs are singing and the heat lightning is beautiful.

My legs still are working enough for me to get up and down and that is HUGE!

Time for sleep, and I'll sleep here with Annie in the den for a while before getting on my "your bed". I do love Annie!

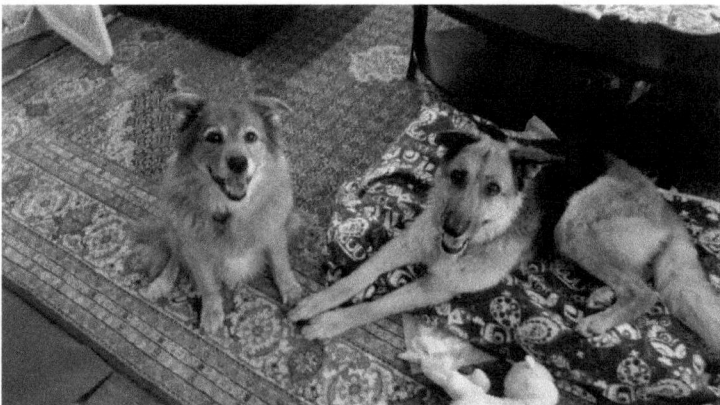

Annie and Sandy

June 23, 2016

I think mom's favorite thing is the cordless vacuum since she likes to use it at least twice a day. She says if she didn't our whole house would have a fur rug. It's been a dark and stormy night with terrible thunder and lightning so we are all hanging close. I do not like thunder! We haven't had to go in the closet yet so that's a good thing. Five animals and two humans in the master closet is not a fun time.

Looks like tomorrow or Saturday will be another bath day. Mom is glad it will only be me and not all three of us. Somehow, in the process of bathing all three of us, mom misplaced (notice I did not say lost) Annie's collar. So last night she decided it might have fallen behind the washer and dryer. So... she pulled the washer and dryer out from the wall and found: two socks, one washcloth, and quite a few Tide pods that had fallen out of the cabinet, and of course, a lot of dust and dog hair. So she cleaned it up and then tried to climb out from behind the narrow space she'd made, ending up having to do the gator across the top of the washer to get out. Silly woman! Doesn't she know 63-year-old women aren't supposed to do stupid things like that? I sure am glad nobody saw her do that! I'd be so embarrassed.

Tonight is a special prayer for all the animals caught in wildfires and floods.

How is it that my mind thinks I'm 33 and I'm having trouble climbing out from behind a washing machine? Another lesson I wasn't prepared for... It would have been an embarrassing situation if I'd had to call for help. I seem to have a knack for doing things that cause me to underestimate my age. I surely wasn't like this at age 30.

June 24, 2016

Yes, Mom found Annie's collar in between the cushion and the side of the chair. I have no earthly idea how it got there!

I haven't had a particularly good day so Mom didn't give me a bath. I threw up all of my breakfast and wet my bed three times today. Mom is suspecting another UTI..... So all my beds now have pads on them and dad is on his third load of wash. I did eat dinner but have tried to eat grass when they take me out so mom gave me some stuff to calm my tummy. Bath tomorrow. Mom and dad already have diapers for me in case this is going to be a persistent problem but we will see how I do tonight.

Thankfully no storms tonight and I'm feeling better after keeping my meds down.

Thank you all for being so supportive and for keeping up with me. You really do keep me and my family going!

June 25, 2016

See, your love and prayers are at work every day! I feel better and didn't wet the beds at all last night or today. I got chicken and rice and coconut oil which is a natural stomach settler. I'm still not quite as energetic as I have been but mom and dad think I'll be back to normal (my normal) by tomorrow. I did enjoy being outdoors several times today and just stood and sniffed the air and listened to the sounds. We had a yellow finch visit today along with our resident mom and dad bluebirds. We had ruby-throated hummingbirds and cardinals! Mom sprayed the crepe myrtle because of those horrible Japanese beetles. Dad mowed and trimmed and Mom weeded.

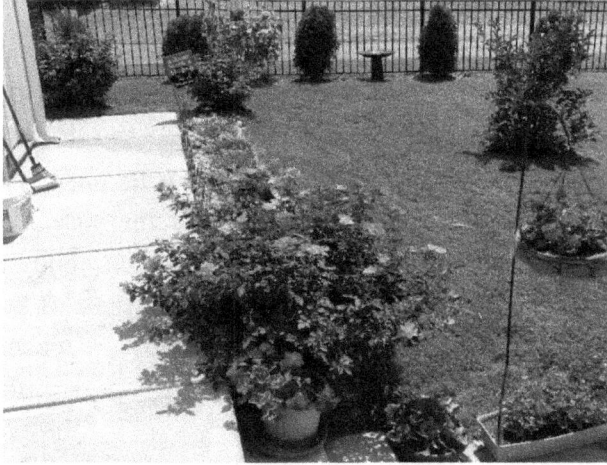

June 26, 2016

Mom had a very busy day because she's helping get a new business location open; she's a consultant and they are opening a new location. I had a walk and I am beyond tired. It's a quiet early night in our household and I'm so thankful for a soft clean "your bed."

Until tomorrow...

June 27, 2016

We have very hot weather right now and so Buddy, Annie and I stay inside most of the time. I'm doing better about drinking water and getting back to my business in the yard. I slept very hard last night and mom put my HEU harness on and I never even woke up. I got up later than usual and my dad got to sleep longer.

I seem a bit weaker in my front legs but I still hold myself up when helped with the harness. Lying on my left side is painful and I cry or whine if my spine gets turned that direction. Mom and dad are calling Dr. Ruth tomorrow to come do some acupuncture and get some pricing. Looks like bath will be on Thursday this week and if it's nice outside I may get to take a bath in the driveway.

One of our kitties is very naughty when she doesn't get a lot of attention. She uses Buddy's bed so mom has to wash it a lot. Buddy's current bed is zillions of cut-up pieces of memory foam in a very flimsy covering that slips into the outside cover. They are so flimsy that she washes them inside a king-size pillowcase. It keeps her from having to pick out all those tiny pieces from the washer and dryer. Lesson learned. Beds are not made to withstand multiple washes. Looking for a new kind.

Here it is the end of June and in January I was destined to be put down. Miracles do happen.

June 29, 2016

Mom thinks the EFAC and the Methyl B12 make a big difference for me so she ordered more. I've received so many wonderful tips on medicines and supplements and something is sure helping.

I can't even begin to tell you about the kindness and graciousness extended to me and my family by my Facebook family. When my folks are tired, you give them strength, when I am having bad days you pray for me and send all that loving energy and if I am not proof of how that works, then nothing is. I know mom looks at so many pups and kitties on a daily basis who are in crisis and our wish tonight is for each of them to have the love and comfort of a family like all of you! Mom says I have taught her to be more patient and more aware of how love works. If we lived on a lot of land, I know we would have a whole pack of dogs and lots of kitties, all of them rescues.

R is for the respite I got when rescued, **E** is for the effort it took Southeast German Shepherd Rescue to save me, **S** is for Sandra, my namesake who helped get me out of the shelter, **C** is for the constant love of my Facebook family, **U** is for the Urgency to save so many more, and **E** is for everyone who steps up to love us and helps us find forever homes.

Our lazy kitty LuLu who is not happy unless she is up on something.

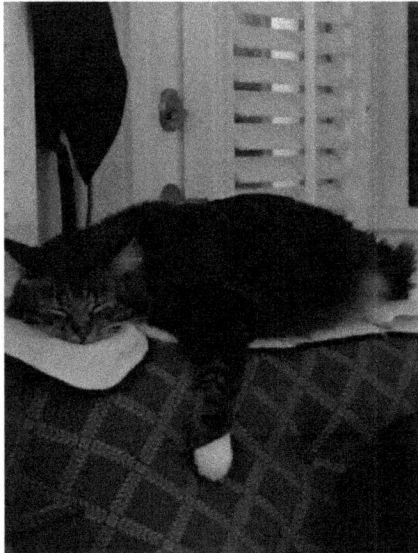

Anyway, today was uneventful other than me bugging Buddy and wanting him to play. He was non-compliant and is just a grouchy old man when I try to play with him. Mom has been working long hours helping get the new shop set up and dad has been taking care of us all day.

So, my next door neighbor has a beautiful Cane Corso they need to re-home. He is black and 3 1/2 years old. The family has an autistic 6-year-old and dad has to travel now with work so two dogs is more than mom has the time to care for, walk, play, etc. since she works long hours too. They are very responsible owners and will require an application process, a meet and greet, and evaluation before rehoming. We are in North Carolina so close to here for a new home would be best. He is as sweet as can be, lives in a fenced yard, has all the inside and outside freedom he wants so that needs to be considered. Mom is helping with this as she has a sharp radar for protecting dogs and putting them in the right homes. I mean, gee, look where I landed!

My human sister has two bully dogs and a toy Aussie so that apple did not fall far from the tree.

We are a fur baby family that's for sure!

June 30, 2016

Stormy night here. Mom worked all day and Dad took care of spraying the yard and plants for Japanese Beetles.

I'm doing the same; no more significant new issues and as active as I can be. I'll be glad when Mom is home more. It's a full-time job to take care of me and all the work is on dad right now.

Sleep well dear friends and say special prayers for the animals caught in the wildfires and floods.

Our motto is "glass half full" and tomorrow, just waking to see the glorious summer is a blessing.

July 2, 2016

I had very sad news today when Mom read through comments from Thursday. A canine police dog named Credo was shot and killed in Long Beach, CA. Do any of you know an organization that raises funds for canine police dogs to have vests that would protect them? If so, please post it... It may be something we can all get behind, and if not, maybe Mom and dad will start a foundation. There isn't a cure for DM but there is a cure for protecting canine police dogs.

Mom and Dad will be leaving music playing or the TV on when leaving the house this weekend. It helps Annie and Buddy and me when all the popping and booming is going on for 4th of July. Have a safe and Happy one!

July 3, 2016

I am fine today and had a nice visit from Peter, Bella, and Bucket.

July 4, 2016

Happy 4th of July. Be safe. Don't do that stupid thing humans do...drink and drive!!!!! Keep your pets where they feel safe through the popping and zinging! Don't leave them outside where noises might make them run in fear.

Love to all my Facebook Family!

I thought it would be another night in the closet with the whole "fam damily," but the fireworks were mild, and we avoided it. I'm putting my tee shirts on them, and that seems to help.

July 5, 2016

Wow, it's been a stormy couple of days here! Mom and Dad went to see the big fireworks. They left the TV on for us but we sure will be glad when they got home! Bella and Peter and Bucket came to visit on Sunday afternoon which our family proclaimed as slug day when we did absolutely nothing but talk and relax. It was a much needed day for Mom after working 7 days straight helping get the new shop open.

Someone in our family (whose initials are Buddy Mahoney) is acting out and decided to use our very nice living room rug a few times, so drastic measures have been taken. Scat mats!!!!! The cats will stop going into that room too. Bahahahaha!

So Mom is investigating area police who have canines to see who might need vests. Somehow she gets herself into having too many irons in the fire...... What's one more!

Special prayers for all the doggies who ran away after being scared by fireworks!

July 7, 2016

You know, with the weather we've been having, it could be the tropics...rain every afternoon, stifling humidity, and bolts upon bolts of lightning! Our potted plants are drowning, so Mom has to drain them!

I must tell you that one of my very kind and generous Facebook friends sent Buddy a new bed (the one the cat used was falling into a zillion pieces) and sent us the coolest inside Chuckit balls and tosser! We all love them and it is so fun for each of us to have one. Thank you from the whole family!

And another loved friend made a donation to the Saving Sandy fund on GoFundMe. My mom and dad are so appreciative and can't tell you how much it has helped us. I go through 28 cans of dog food a week... I don't eat grains so if anyone has any cost-saving advice on dog food please, please send it!

Tomorrow is a walk day in the morning before the rain comes. I had a delightful bath today!!!

<u>Note from Mom</u>

As I am proofing this book, it comes to mind that here, years later, our new GSD rescue has a favorite toy in the yard. It is the Chuckit ball sent by Sandy's friend! Ragged and chewed, it has lasted these years and has been passed on to another rescue pup.

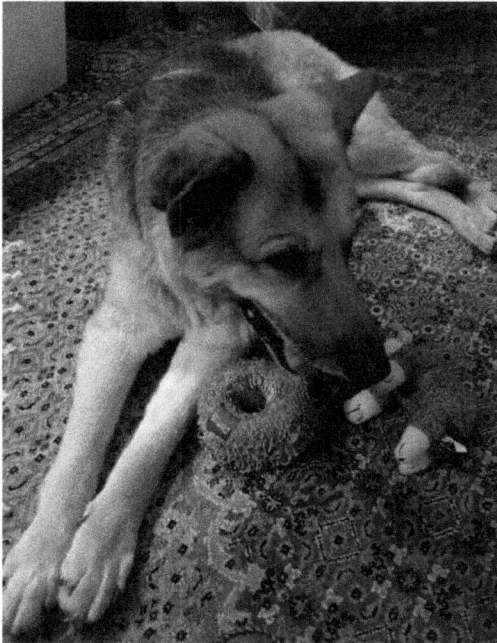

July 8, 2016

Mom has been trying to figure out how to make an Amazon wish list get to my page, which is a page from her personal Facebook page, so if she shares the list, it goes to her personal page, not mine. All hints are welcome!!!

I've gotten so tired of lying on my right side and it hurts me to lie on my left side. Mom is calling Dr. Ruth tomorrow. I'm whining a lot now especially in the evening. So if any of you know of a natural muscle relaxer or supplement that helps with this, please let me know..... Oh, and please remember to share my posts so we reach a lot of people dealing with Degenerative Myelopathy.

Dr. Ruth West is coming to see me next Saturday! I'm soooo glad! In the meantime, Mom is getting some turmeric and I got a 45-minute massage tonight. I loved it! Then I got brushed all over and it felt wonderful. So I will get one daily now and tomorrow we will go for a short walk! Mom will work on a wish list over the weekend since some of you have requested one. Going in the water may be a challenge getting me to the lake but we will look into it. I actually enjoyed my warm shower the other day.

Pray tonight and tomorrow and the days after for love and peace. Remember that no one is promised tomorrow, it is but a gift! Each one of us can light a candle in our hearts for hatred to not be a part of our own little corner of the world. Our love to all of you. You matter.

July 10, 2016

I got another massage today but didn't have a very good appetite. But my nose is cool and all else normal so Mom and Dad aren't worrying. Tomorrow is the day for Mom to work on the wish list.

The horrible blood shedding is not only in the dog fighting world and the world of cruelty to dogs but is now brewing among humans. The difference is that humans have a choice.

I am on my left side and made the decision all by myself. I got my massage and I just was so sore on my right side that I finally gave in to being on my left side. It's been a long day and my legs aren't very strong today. My water intake is down and hopefully, I'll be better tomorrow. Mom is hoping I will sleep on my left side all night.

What a roller coaster ride this is.

July 11, 2016

I'm drinking my water and eating normally..... My back legs are just weaker. Mom and Dad put me in my wheels, and we walked around the corner and back. It was a big journey for me. I'm worn out..... And back on my right side but at least my back was exercised a bit. The spondylosis is bad in my lower spine but making myself move around keeps me from being so stiff. The light is still in my eyes, and today was better than yesterday........ Once again, the power of prayer. You know, people could learn a lot from dogs about getting along and caring for one another.

July 12, 2016

Mom will work on the wish list, but right now, my biggest wish is for acupuncture more often. My spine is getting more crooked and we are all anxiously awaiting Dr. Ruth on Saturday. We don't know yet what it will cost to have her come but Mom and Dad will get her as often as possible. I've gotten quite good at falling onto my right side in order to lie down or when I come in on the harness and go to get in my bed. This means that I swing my butt around to the right as hard as I can and throw myself down on my "your bed". I missed the bed today and landed on Annie. She wasn't happy about it.

And now to our fallen policemen: better love hath no man than he who lays down his life for another. Pass it on and pay it forward

July 13, 2016

It's unbelievable! I will get to have multiple acupuncture sessions and Mom and Dad will take me for more laser therapy! It's overwhelming and I just pray the people who are working to wipe out animal cruelty and neglect and abuse know they are angels. I was within hours of being euthanized now I am loved and cared for and hopeful that one day no more pups will suffer from DM. American Kennel Club should require reporting DM in a bloodline!!!!

Note From Mom

As of the date of this publishing, it is known that there is a genetic predisposition to DM but that other factors most likely contribute. Testing is recommended by the AKC but not required. For further information, go to Infographic - Quick Facts on Degenerative Myelopathy and Genetic Testing - New Research - DogWellNet

July 15, 2016

All is ok. Don't worry. Mom had a busy day and late night on a goodwill mission. More tomorrow, so rest well. I'm already on my "your bed."

I was an early riser this morning because Mom had to be gone by 8:15...... and somehow in the rush, I didn't get my breakfast ...... and Mom and Dad felt really badly when they fed me early afternoon, so I got special treatment!

Mom says I am such a good girl and so smart; it makes her mad that someone didn't teach me all the manners and commands because I learn so quickly. However, I can be somewhat strong-willed and that's probably why I'm still here.

Dr. Ruth West comes tomorrow for my acupuncture! It's very exciting and I am such a lucky girl to be able to have the treatment.

Please pray tonight for humans who are grieving and for humans who don't understand grace.

July 16, 2016

Oh I had the nicest acupuncture treatment from Dr. Ruth!!!! I've been so relaxed that even the horrible thunder storms haven't bothered me much. We did have a bad one where there was talk of everyone moving into the master bedroom closet..... But we didn't have to go. I'll have another treatment on the 29th!

Lately here, we seem to have bad thunder storms almost every night. It's sort of like the tropics, Mom says, but it doesn't pass over as fast.

I hear Mom and Dad talking all about this thing called an election. From what I make of it all, it is humans being as nasty and mean, deceitful and bragging...... I don't get it. You know, dogs do a lot of listening... And most of us are pretty good at it. But we do a lot of speaking too, by speaking from our hearts and souls. I think people could learn a lot by listening to dogs more than they do political talk.

Hoping for people to open their hearts along with their eyes and ears because they are the ones who have choices, not us.

<u>July 18, 2016</u>

It's getting close to bedtime here at our house, and we've all had our trip outside and been given our nightly treats. My mom and dad love us so much and even though our house seems to grow hair every day and we go through vacuum bags like crazy, and even though we have yoga mats stretched from rug to rug, we are all so blessed to live in a home full of love. It seems this country has gone crazy so much of the time and it's comforting to know that home is a safe place and a good place.

Prayer of St. Francis of Assisi:

Lord, make me an instrument of thy peace

Where there is hatred, let me sow love

Where there is injury, pardon

Where there is discord, union

Where there is error, truth

Where there is doubt, faith

Where there is despair, hope

Where there is darkness, light

Where there is sadness, joy

O Master, let me not seek as much to be consoled as to

console

To be understood, as to understand

To be loved as to love.

For it is in giving that one receives.

It is in pardoning that one is pardoned

It is in dying that one is raised to eternal life

La Ligue de la Sainte-Messe

July 19, 2016

Thanks to all the love and care from my extended family, I remain on a special diet designed to help me with maintaining a steady weight but rich in nutrition......it is VERY tasty! Now..... Buddy and Annie have caught on that mine smells better than theirs, so if we get fed at the same time, they lurk around me and my bowl for any micro speck of food I might drop. They lurk while their food lies waiting in their bowls in the laundry room and only go eat their own when all chances of spare morsels from mine fade away. Now, Mom and Dad have gotten on to their lurking so I usually get fed after they eat. I may be slow and creaky but I'm not stupid! So I make sure I eat all my food.

Today was good because I still got around on the carpet and am able to go out with help.

Bless the men in Blue, dear God

Keep them safe and strong.

Help us to understand they cannot be policemen and teachers and counselors and missionaries to the communities and still be good husbands and fathers on the very little pay we allow them to be paid.

Help us search our souls to understand they can't rescue all the abused and neglected pets while humans are busy killing each other. Help us help them by expecting more of ourselves. Be strong and of good courage!

July 21, 2016

I heard a story today about another dog who died from being left in the heat. It took a piece of my heart. How can human beings be deemed the most intelligent inhabitants of the earth and use their positions of dominion so poorly?

What must a neglected and abused animal feel in those horrible moments?

Well...I can tell you a little about this and ask each of you to share my posts and my page with the public.

You first begin to realize that something is not right when your stomach is empty, and hunger pains strike, or when that broomstick hits you in the head and over your back, or when the full force of being kicked in the ribs throws you against the ground. Your head drops and you wonder what you did to deserve this from your human. Then you realize that even though the rain has soaked through your fur, and there is nothing but mud at the end of your chain, there is little hope, and your eyes begin to become vacant and your head drops lower. You begin to be afraid when you hear someone approaching, but you hope against hope that they might take mercy and throw you a morsel, a cracker, molded bread... Anything... And you begin to cower down and curl up in a ball as you shiver from fright.

And for a few of us, that sound has turned out to be the footsteps of a rescuer, and we go haltingly and shaking, with a tiny spark of hope in our heart that the ride we are taking is a ride to safety.

We are all worn out and ready for bed. It has been a quiet day watching Mom do chores and we enjoyed napping. The veterinary school of medicine called today to check on how I am doing. They were so kind to me when I was there!

Many of you send such wonderful messages to me and make comments. We try to read every one of them, and they are the prayers that nurture us every day. The power of love is proven

I hope that if you take anything away from this story, it is the story of the horrible abuse of animals by people. Every letter, every email, every dime you can send, and every animal you can foster, helps build the case to prosecute these horrible people.

July 22, 2016

My mom's sister is also a rescuer of German Shepherds and kitties and bunnies and birds and on and on. They have a tradition that they quietly do whenever one of their fur babies crosses the rainbow bridge. Before the sister who has lost a pet can notice, the other sister has quietly removed the bowls, the toys, the bed of the pet who has crossed and placed them carefully out of sight until the pain has subsided a bit. Anyway, for my mom's birthday (which was a month ago), my auntie gave my mom a beautiful piece pictured below. It's too perfect. And each time she sees it, she remembers Tammy, Maggie, India, Cubby, Sasha, Kittyboo, Mollie, Gammon, Ladybug, Nimh, Morris, Simone, Noodle, Boots, Casey, Katie, Pandy, Micky, Bama, all...pieces of their hearts and parts of the decades of their lives. All of them contributing to the kind of people they are today. Blessed to have loved them.

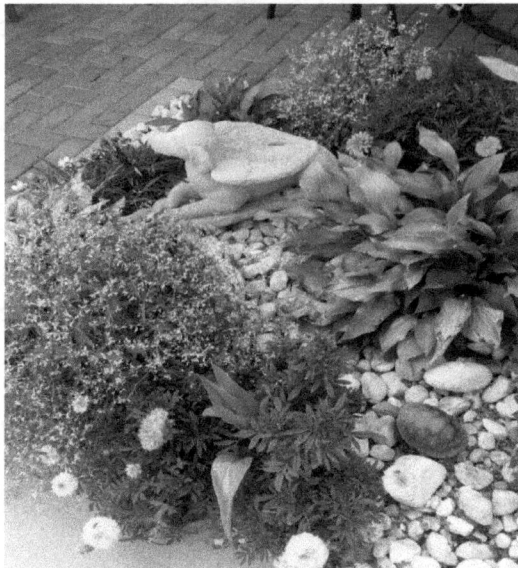

July 24, 2016

Well...The brood is here, so I feel like I'm in a pack of hoodlums! Peter and Bella bark at people who walk down the alley and then Bucket starts in and then Annie and Buddy, and it's a crazy place!

Our neighbors are all scared of Bella and Peter, which is hilarious because they are both scaredy cats! It was so awfully hot today that they got cabin fever and made me a little crazy. However, a big move for me: I shoved Peter around a bit and wouldn't let him lie next to my dad!!! Ha ha ha!

We are in for some scorchers, so tell all your friends to make sure their pets are inside and have lots of water! Be on the lookout for strays who need water, and try to carry some take-out containers in your car with bottled water in case you see dogs and cats suffering from heat.

I've stayed pretty busy today trying to make sure I move myself closer to Mom or Dad than Peter or Bella. I did play with Peter a bit today, and Annie must have thought he was trying to hurt me because she came right up and gave him a piece of her mind!!!! Poor Peter wouldn't hurt a flea and is still so young and playful. The good news is that he wore me out, and all the positioning has made me tired. Mom decided to move two large Hosta today as the sun was going down and they were in a spot that was burning them up. Not the best timing in the world... Like maybe it should have been done a month ago, but it got done. Dad spent two hours watering, and tomorrow is supposed to be as hot as today. But we do have three tomatoes that are almost ripe!

We continue to read so much information on DM and Mom is convinced the supplements I get are key to my still being able to stand. That and all the power of prayer and loving energy that you send me every day. It is hard to put into words the feeling that comes over us when we realize that six and a half months ago, I was scheduled to be euthanized because no one wanted me. I think of all the pups who are scheduled for tomorrow and pray that one day we will have no more homeless dogs or cats.

July 25, 2016

Some of my Facebook family has asked for my list of meds and supplements. We've tried many things but have settled into these that have kept me on my legs for four months now:

Dasaquin

EFAC - ordered on Amazon

VitaLife - multivitamins

Methyl B12- Costco or Amazon

Fish Oil

Pure Frankincense oil in diffuser mist

My meds:

Tramadol

Gabapentin

Rimadyl

My food:

Grain-free canned food mixed with Primal Patties plus 1 Tbl. Coconut oil

Weekly or every other week acupuncture

Daily massage

July 26, 2016

Thank goodness we had a thunderstorm tonight and the plants got some water. Along with a lot of the country, we are having major hot days.... Brutal to us fur babies if we are out too long. I've spent the day lounging in the cool of the air conditioning and feeling so blessed to have a soft bed and AC and water. I am living the good life and just want to work hard to help homeless pups and kitties and make humans aware of their responsibilities that come with having dominion over all things.

I would also like to ask each of you to also follow the Degenerative Myelopathy Facebook page. It is really informative but is also another chance for you to send love and healing to pups in need.

Mom's Frankenstein boot is not slowing her down much. She says her foot doesn't hurt when in the boot, so that's a good thing, and all she is taking is Advil. She says to thank you all for the good wishes and prayers but she's one tough cookie and hates to be held back. She's also very hard-headed and stubborn like me. It's a real inconvenience to her, that's all.

Drink water, stay calm, and don't get overheated.

July 28, 2016

No worries. I fell asleep early last night and so did Mom. More tonight, and have a cool day!

A reflection on what really is important from my perspective (thoughts inspired by the political hatred, viciousness, vitriol, lying, accusations, and complete utter negativity):

It is important that I have love from my family and that I love my family.

I live in a country that doesn't eat dogs.

I have a family who is free to give me shelter and a home where I am safe.

I don't live on a concrete floor or a dirt yard.

I don't have chains on me.

I love my kitties, the sunshine and even the rain.

I love breathing fresh air.

My heart is healed every day by friends.

My tummy is full and I have all the clean water I want.

I have the medicine I need.

I live each day the best way I can.

I believe in the power of prayer and healing energy.

I have a soft place to sleep.

I get kisses on the top of my head.

I get lots of encouragement.

I give away as much love as I take.

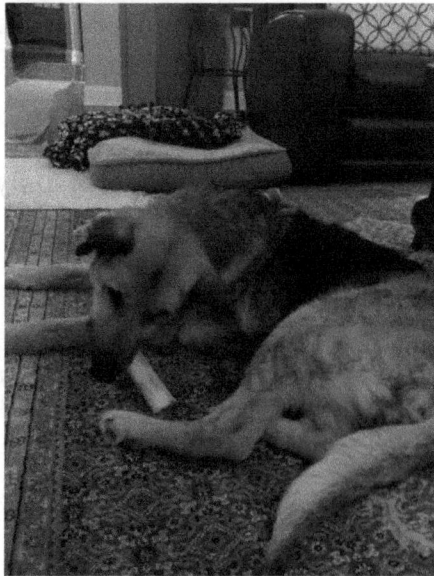

July 29, 2016

The sun rose and the day began with my breakfast and a visit from Dr. Ruth West who did acupuncture and electrotherapy. It was FABULOUS. Mom put on soft classical music and I enjoyed the session while on my "your bed."

I slept most of the afternoon and have been so relaxed and happy that I've even wagged my tail over dinner and meeting Mom and Dad at the door when they came in from working in the yard. Life is good. Bad hind legs will not keep my spirits down.

My next-door neighbor, Ajax, is still looking for a loving home. He's a sweet boy, and please send positive thoughts for him.

And when you go to bed tonight, close your eyes tightly and be thankful for the United States of America. One nation under God, with liberty and justice for all we were, and with hope, we will be again.

July 30, 2016

The heat has kept me inside more than usual and I'm getting bored lying around. So tomorrow, after the hot sun begins to set, my mom and dad are taking the three of us to the lake. It's going to be a big undertaking so pray it goes well for us. Mom and Dad re-landscaped the side of the patio today in 102 degrees. They are either crazy or trying to have heart attacks. Anyway, it got done.

Some things I wonder about:

Do the animals in the forest get afraid of thunder like I do?

Do Annie and Buddy know I can't use my legs very well?

How will the birds we feed ever know not to be afraid in our yard?

How does my tail wag sometimes and not others?

Silly things.... Yet nice to wonder and I really don't need the answers. We are all just where we are; it's what we do with being where we are that counts.

July 31, 2016

Well, the rain and storms kept us from the lake today and Mom was disappointed. It's supposed to rain tomorrow too but if it's clear and cool enough, we will go then to the lake. I didn't have a great day... The down side of the roller coaster. My legs were weaker today, and I wet my bed. So Mom will keep an eye out for possible bladder infection, and Mom and Dad will give me all the help I need to go out.

Thunder and lightning here, but we need the rain. And yes to our friend Rex... I do think it's time for another garlic and bologna sandwich.

We have hummingbirds who come every morning and every late afternoon, and tomorrow Mom will send a picture of the sunflowers that the birds planted.

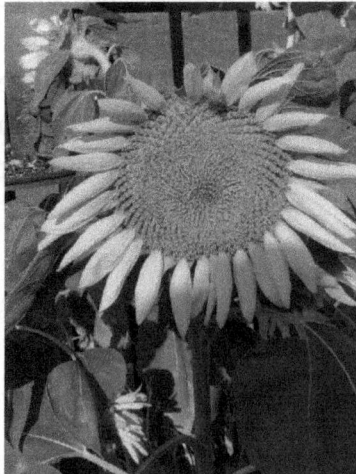

August 2, 2016

Today was a bit better but I am whining tonight. Prayers work!!!!! Mom and Dad send their deep appreciation for all the encouragement!

And now abides faith, hope, and love. But the greatest of these is love.
1 Corinthians 13:13

Sleep well. Mom and I fell asleep early, and I didn't update my posts. So sorry! Anyway, yesterday Mom got the nicest get-well card from one of my Facebook friends. She was very touched.

I am having more difficulty with my back legs and not getting around like I did last week. We are hoping it is just the down hill of the roller coaster, and I will be moving around better in a few days. In the meantime, keep me in your thoughts and prayers, and thank you!

August 4, 2016

Oh my! We all were asleep on the sofa last night ....it was a very early morning yesterday! But oh wow do prayer work! I feel so much better today and have been able to get up on my own all day long! It's exciting for me and I get all fired up and try to get Annie to play while Mom and Dad just smile ear to ear. I had a pretty remarkable day and you will never be able to tell me that prayers don't work!!!!! Thank you for each and every prayer and all the love. You are keeping me able to enjoy life!

Mom has a torn tendon in her left foot. Which means..... either learn to deal with discomfort (which is her preference) or surgery which she hates! Nevertheless, the boot is still in use for a little bit.

We haven't made it to the lake yet but if I am the same tomorrow, we will try to go.

We are all sending each of you much love and great appreciation for your prayers and your loyalty..... If you have a moment, please pray for Augustus. He is a very sick dog who was rescued by Trio Animal Foundation. He was starving and suffering from a bullet wound. He needs the power of your love.

August 5, 2016

And.... I had another good day and I started it off very early. Woke Dad about 4:00 am so I could go out. Dad was so sleepy but so happy I can still know when I need to go out. So I got breakfast at 6:00 a.m. because I decided to stand at the bedroom door and pant. I've been pretty active (well, active for me) today. Tonight I even got up and went across the room to get my tennis ball, and brought it back to show it to Mom. She got the hint.

I have begged and begged Buddy to play and he won't. I even took myself to my "your bed" in the bedroom for a nap!

You are all so wonderful to stay in touch with me, and after so many months, you are all still so loyal and so devoted to pray for me and send me healing love.

Augustus is in intensive care. He has burns and sores and a bullet wound and looks like a skeleton but he wagged his skinny tail today when caregivers came to feed him. Trio Animal Foundation works miracles every day. We follow them, among many other rescues, but this guy really touched my heart, and that's why I think it's so important to let you know about him.

August 6, 2016

I am putting up pictures to show how prayers and healing works. Mom and Dad are humbled by your power and by the love they experience through you. I am thankful for each day I can be happy and each time I can lie on my "your bed." I am thankful......we are thankful.

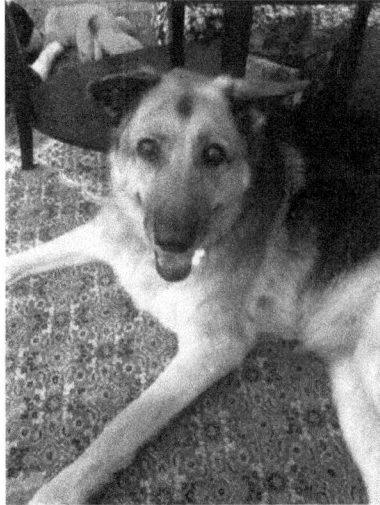

August 7, 2016

Isn't it wonderful? I am still pulling myself around and going to my other bed in the master bedroom whenever I want to. It's been happy days, and all of us are so thankful! I am a very smart girl too, and have the bedtime treat routine down to a science. I still like to get Dad up at 6:00...he's not too fond of that and wishes Mom would wake up when I start panting.

Off to watch Olympics and swimming...Mom's favorite.

August 8, 2016

We have had a pretty stormy day but I am still doing well. I got up this morning and demanded to be fed....so my day began early. Then Mom went with my human sister to look at a new equestrian place. I'm pretty tired tonight and will take myself to bed in a few minutes. (I love being able to do that!! I started it last week and when I feel sleepy. I just get up and wobble into the bedroom).

Many have asked for updates on Augustus. I want you to know that we made a donation to him from my GoFundMe account ...A small one but we couldn't not help. Anyway, here is the latest from their Facebook page

AUGUSTUS UPDATE 8/8/16 1:58 pm: We are so happy to report that Augustus no longer has diarrhea. We believe that the combination of traditional medicine with a homeopathic approach is working to improve his condition and heal him from the inside out.

Augustus continues to receive silver sulfadiazine treatments along with chlorhexidine scrubs on both lesions. The lesion from the gunshot wound has been healing very well and is almost fully granulated with new, healthy tissue. The pressure wound has also filled in with healthy tissue as well, but it still has a way to go before it is fully healed.

For the next 10 days, Augustus will continue on his oral antibiotics, pain meds and supplements. After that, his medical team will recheck his bloodwork to determine if his infections have resolved with the antibiotics.

He seems much more alert and bright, which is truly heartwarming to see. You can even see a little tail wag in his photo!

Please continue to keep Augustus in your thoughts and prayers. We truly believe that it has helped in his recovery. Also, thank you so

much to everybody who is helping TAF to get Augustus the best medical care possible. This is truly a team effort, and he is counting on all of us!

August 9, 2016

Please pray hard for what is best for Augustus. He has taken a bad turn, and we want to focus our energies and thoughts and prayers on him tonight. He needs your energies and love. We are sending ours to him.

He is back in ICU and they are working desperately to help him.

I am dealing with a lack of appetite and a little diarrhea but it may be because I'm sharing Mom and Dad's attention....... Bella and Bucket are here. No need to worry. I went into the kitchen when Mom was fixing dinner, so I do have an appetite, just maybe not for dog food. Hahahahaha.

One of the reasons we are posting about Augustus is because Trio Animal Foundation takes in the very worst cases of abuse and neglect and is so extremely focused on what is best for each and every one they bring in. They help when no one else can. They saved little Hazel Grace when she had been held over a gas burner and so many more. We are lifting prayers up tonight because Augustus needs us so much.

August 11, 2016

All is ok here. I'm so tired from keeping up with Bella that I am going to sleep on my left side!

First time in a few weeks.

Augustus is still in ICU. Lots of people are working to save him, including all of my Facebook family.

His eye is on the sparrow!

August 13, 2016

Mom and Dad decided rather be safe than sorry, so off to the vet, I went about my diarrhea. Had tests run on my counts, so no bacteria and no urinary tract infection; however, hahaha, I do get chicken and rice for a few days. Mom boiled 10 chicken thighs, skinned them and added them to a big pot of rice. I loved my dinner!!!!!! It is stressful to go to the vet for me so tonight I've been sleeping a lot. Dad is hoping I won't get him up in another hour.

So, I'm off to the land of nod and will post more tomorrow. Thank you for all the prayers and best wishes. I am beating the odds one day at a time.

August 14, 2016

Oh today was lazy!!!! It's way too hot and humid to be outside long and we are so thankful for air conditioning! I'm loving my chicken and rice! Will probably be adding some sweet potato gradually.It's late and last night I got Mom up at 2:00 and again at 7:00 so we are going to say prayers and send thanks for today and yesterday! Blessings to all of you, my wonderful family!

I am amazing my mom and dad with my independence indoors. They seem to be quite amused at my taking myself to bed and wanting to have part of their dinner. I don't get their dinner. But am taking myself to bed and lying in my left side. Tummy is settled down too!

I have a very special request for a special two-legged friend who is going through a loss. Could I impose on you to say a prayer for my friend. Your love and prayers are so powerful, and we never take them for granted. In fact, your prayers and healing thoughts and energies have healed all of us in so many ways. Our faith has been reinforced and you have held us up on many hard days.

We are so thankful for this circle of friends on this earth who have connected through your love for me. We are so, so blessed. So here is a thank you picture from us

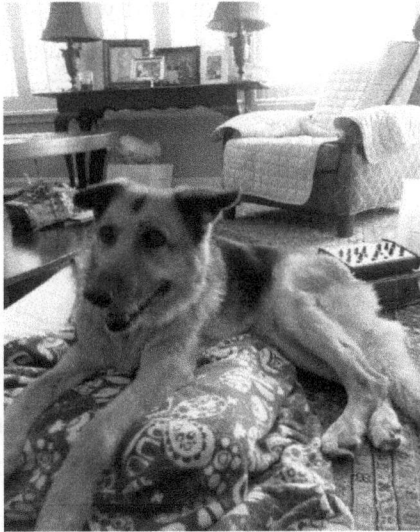

August 15, 2016

We have a very special need tonight. One of my Facebook family has found out that this adorable GSD needs a new home. His people are moving and cannot take him. He is reasonably close to us in location and thorough checking of any potential new homes will be done.

Please share this news with only loving animal people as we must protect him from anyone who would not be a good owner. Private message me if you want more info.

August 17, 2016

We are so happy to let you know the 7-month-old GSD pup has a wonderful new home and our deepest thanks for all your prayers and efforts on his behalf. I had a better day today than yesterday. Mom tried to trim my nails and she felt so guilty about cutting one too close that she couldn't even let me tell you about it last night. It was awful. It hurt me and I panicked, and of course, we had blood all over me, all over Mom, all over the oriental rug and all over Dad because I wouldn't let them keep a towel around my foot and it took 30 minutes to stop. It looked like a horror show but we got it all cleaned up and I am fine now. Mom is still freaked out. Yes, we have a Drimmel but I hate that buzzy thing........ However, Mom won't be doing that again. Maybe Dr. RUTH CAN HELP WHEN SHE COMES.

August 17, 2016

Today was house cleaning day so we spent a lot of time avoiding the vacuum and the floor cleaner. They make soooo much noise.

An update on Augustus; he has another medical emergency tonight with a terribly swollen neck and side of his face. Trio Animal Foundation is still working to help him and he is in the best possible hands for any help that is possible. Pray for his comfort and the wisdom of his caregivers. Thanks so much for sharing your love with him.

I have already taken myself to bed.

August 19, 2016

Well we all got Mom up at 6:45 a.m. acting like idiots. Panting and prancing and whining... so out we went outside with the sole intention of browsing around the yard...

Bella loves to try to chase Tipper and Lulu but she gets a very scary voice from Mom when she tries. Somehow in the goings on yesterday, Mom left her car door slightly open, so today, when she went to go out, her battery was slightly DEAD. Triple AAA to the rescue along with Dad's best bud Kevin. All was not lost. We still got groceries which is more than those poor souls in Louisiana have right now. Mom wishes she could join a rescue group to go help.

We are all pretty blest here at Austin Creek. We all have beds and grass and meals and treats, and for the most part, the rest of the crew are all healthy. A good day to be thankful for our abundance and our health. Mom was one of those cheerleaders who married the big football player and now they spend their time loving us and making sure we are all ok. They are pretty young for 63 and we all love them so much. We are all spoiled rotten and only get the best so we know we are blessed beyond belief.

Pass a blessing on to an animal tomorrow. A pat on the head, a fresh bowl of water, a cup of ice cubes, carry sunscreen to put on a white dog's nose or ears, just anything to pay it forward to another dog or cat tomorrow.

Ok I fell asleep before I finished the post and now it's in the stratosphere somewhere. So don't worry, I'll write more tonight but have a good Friday all my FB Family. You are all very powerful people!!!! I am evidence.

Bella has pulled all the toys out of the toy box and we are lying side by side, having a good old toy fest.

We had some thunder and hard rain but it has passed for now so we are happy babies. Annie and Buddy and Bucket are asleep.

Mom had a very early morning and dad slept in...Mom had to work today so dad took care of the yard and sprayed for mosquitos. Both

Kim and dad got eaten by them yesterday because they are too hard-headed about bug spray.

I'm a bit tired on my feet today from all the trying to keep up with blocking Bella.

Time for Mom to order more Methyl B12 and my EFAC. The prayers you send are miracle workers for me and I am so grateful for all of you my family.

Looking back, there are so many times when I wish I would have taken pictures. I was so involved in being beside Sandy that I never even thought of getting the camera.

August 20, 2016

For my new Facebook Friends (with love and gratitude to my loyal friends since January!!):

I was to be euthanized in 24 hours when Southeast German Shepherd Rescue called my mom at 7:00 in the evening on a January Tuesday. They needed a foster family to commit to take me before they could pull me from the shelter. I had been severely abused and neglected. So Mom went home from rehearsal to talk to Dad about saving me. They already had two dogs who were both rescued, and two rescued cats so really weren't looking for another 4-legged child. They are both huge animal lovers, so they called Southeast German Shepherd Rescue Wednesday morning just in time to keep me from being euthanized, and said they would foster me. Twenty-four hours later, I was in a veterinary office when my foster mom and dad arrived. I was covered in démodectic mange, I had no hair on my tail or neck or chest or stomach and no hair on my back except black fuzz where my saddle marks are. My nails were at least 4 inches long and I could not stand up. I smelled horrible and had pus coming out of my right ear. They took me home and I actually had a bed and a blanket and food and water and medicine to help me get better. I had to be bathed twice a week in the big glass box my mom calls a shower and I only weighed 56 pounds.

So to make a long story a bit shorter, Mom and Dad adopted me. My medical needs are always going to be pretty extensive so at the request of many Facebook friends, my mom put up a GoFundMe page. Because of that, I now have custom-made wheels and all my meds, and I also get physical therapy and acupuncture every two weeks. I was diagnosed as having Degenerative Myelopathy and severe spondylosis but with my mom's and dad's persistence and love, I am still able to wobble around on all four legs, as long as there is grass or carpet or yoga mats (which appear in many places in our house!) I have to have help to hold myself up to go to the bathroom but I have ramps to use to get up and down into the yard, so my Ginger harness and my Help Em Up Harness are always in use. I have a brother, Buddy, and a sister, Annie, and two kitties, Tipper and Lulu. Bella and Bucket are my human sister's four-legged children, and they come stay with us a lot because she travels for her job. I have a bed in the den and a bed in the bedroom and I have my fur back. I love my toys and cannot believe that my days of hoping when I was wet and cold, I was hurting, and so sad...those days are gone. We, as a family, work hard to spread the word about abuse and neglect of animals and about things that help with degenerative myelopathy. I appreciate every meal, very soft caress, every happy moment because of the prayers and positive healing energies thousands have sent to me on my page.

So enough for tonight, and for tomorrow, welcome the new day, say a kind word, and help an animal who needs it, even if you are just sharing a post on Facebook.

August 21, 2016

It's a quiet night and I am exhausted after doing my best for a week to keep up with Bella. She's at home with her mom now along with Bucket, and I am in my "your bed" (Mom washed it today, so everything is fluffy and fresh).

For my friends who ask about Augustus, he's had a setback but has an extreme will to live. Your prayers for him gets him through the week, so please keep up the good work and thank you for every single word you've said and every single prayer you've made and every single thought you've had on my behalf. I am living proof that prayer, love, and hope works!

You can follow Augustus on Trio Animal Foundation's Facebook page. That's what we do.

August 25, 2016

Down for the evening. I had a wonderful acupuncture session today and I've been so relaxed all day I have barely gotten up.

Bella and Bucket come back tomorrow night so it will be a busy weekend.

Augustus made a tiny bit of progress today so that's a good thing.

Blessings to all this late evening and a bright morning to you when you awake.

August 26, 2016

No worries. Dad and I are hanging out with Annie, Buddy, Bella and Bucket while Mom visits her best friends. We've kept dad on his toes and tried to be good company to him. He's not as mushy as Mom so we sometimes have to be rather insistent either "pay attention to ME" gestures. He's a good dad to be so helpful with all of us.

Not much news... Except that another pretty good day is pretty big news. Thank all of you for what you do for me and the encouragement every day. I am so blessed to have all of you!

August 29 2016

Let's get caught up. Mom went to have a few days with her best friends of 45 years and Dad had to take care of all five of us. We all survived and everything is back to normal. Bella and Bucket went back home last night and we are all in our normal spots tonight.

I'm still wobbling around on the carpet and needing help to hold myself up outside but am glad things haven't progressed any further. I had a wonderful acupuncture session on this last Wednesday and I'm back to doing my best to be a dog.

I am teaching my parents more every day about German Shepherds and our ways. They get amused when I get so possessive. But there's a lot of love in this house and more than enough to go around.

We all send our love and blessings to you, my family, and promise to be better about pictures.

August 30, 2016

Reflecting on today:

I slept until 7:00 a.m., a banner event in our household.

I immediately got breakfast after going out first thing!

I proceeded to go back to sleep while Mom could not....

Mom worked today and Dad did yard stuff while we all tried to go in and out as much as possible.

We got a good report on Augustus that he's making progress.

I took great interest in the toad that lives somewhere near our rock garden until he jumped and I almost fell down.

And now it's bed time and I get treats now.

There was a report on the news about how dogs know what their parents are saying to them, and I can't figure out why that is news because anyone with a dog already knows this......

Mom had rehearsal tonight, first of the fall season, and wouldn't share the pizza when she got home.

September 1, 2016

So here's how I figure miracles work:

A policeman noticed me in a very bad place in very bad condition and he took me to a shelter.

In the shelter, a kind woman named Sandra just knew in her heart I deserved a chance.

She contacted a rescue organization.

The rescue organization had my mom and dad's information because they had made a donation previously to honor a member of their family.

They called my mom and dad in urgent need of a foster family for me so I would not be euthanized.

My mom and dad picked me up from the rescue and nursed me 24/7 because I was so completely at rock bottom.

My mom decided more people needed to be fosters and to know about dogs like me, so she started my Facebook page

All of you began one by one to follow me and my family grew to thousands

Some of you encouraged Mom and Dad to start a GoFundMe account since my medical care was going to cost a huge amount of money.

Mom had to think about it for a while, but you convinced her.

And you sent me life-saving gifts, blankets, bed, toys, supplements and treats.

You sent me to North Carolina State University Veterinary School of Medicine where they could diagnose me.

You sent me therapy; hydrotherapy, laser therapy, acupuncture and physical therapy.

I began to walk.

You suggested supplements to try, and we did.

8 months later, I am still able to walk, even if wobbly and not far.

I now love to be in the center of things, and I love having water and food and a bed.

Most of all, I love having you as my family and having a real mom and dad.

If you don't believe in miracles, look at each sentence above. Every single one is a miracle!

PS: Mom says to tell you we also watch Hillary as well as Donald. We aren't happy with either of them.

So tonight, say prayers for our country and for wisdom.

My dad was a 32nd Degree Mason and was the most honorable man I've ever known. I inherited one of his Bibles, and throughout it, he has circled or marked the word wisdom. We can all strive to be wise. In the coming in, and in the going out, in the living and the dying, and in knowing our path.

September 3, 2016

My cousins are visiting, and I do so love these little girls!!!!!! They are kind and sweet to me, and I love their hugs!

Your messages made my mom teary-eyed for the outpouring of love.

Isn't it such a message that a tiny woman who spent her life helping the neglected and poor and sick will now be made a Saint, while we as a nation struggle between voting for one of two people who are both the antithesis of Mother Teresa......

God help us.

Each of us must keep the hope alive, we must love and care for all God's creatures, even if it is in our own tiny little spot on this earth. Our journey depends on the roads we choose, according to my mom and dad. We choose the road of hope, love, forgiveness, and integrity. We are so blessed to have you with us on this journey!

September 4, 2016

Are you ready for some fooooootballll? If not, you wouldn't like it at our house! (Mom rolls her eyes here).

We escaped the brunt of the tropical storm Hermine and had a gorgeous day today. I loved my little girls but they returned home so now Bella and Bucket are back because their mom is traveling. I get good mental and physical stimulation with Bella here, because it's my job to make sure she doesn't overstep her bounds with Mom and Dad.

Somehow someone in our neighborhood failed to remember that this is Labor Day weekend and NOT July 4th. The booming and popping of fireworks has made me just about crazy and Bella has barked so much that Mom finally really fussed at her. Glad it wasn't me because after that fussing, I don't want to be on the receiving end of it ever!

Lulu and Tipper retreat to the upstairs when Bella is here because Bella will chase them. They run, Bella chases, Mom fusses. I think Bella needs to have a good cat scratch!

If you are anywhere near the coastal areas that got hit and can possibly foster a lost cat or dog or baby squirrel that fell out of a tree, please let your local shelters know!

September 7, 2016

Had my last acupuncture today for a while thanks to a wonderful gift of sessions from a member of my Facebook. I have amazed everyone and am still able to stand (not long) and eat and enjoy life. I will sleep like a rock tonight, and Mom and Dad hope to be able to schedule some sessions in a couple of weeks. Annie is asleep beside me and she really does a good job staying close by me. Mom and Dad continue with my regimen and swear it's the right mix to keep me moving around.

Who knew that I'd be a happy permanent member of the Mahoney family when I came here in January. It's all a miracle.

September 8, 2016

We are so thankful because each person who reads about me lifts me up in spirit and I continue to be happy. My legs are wobbly and numb but they are perfect. My skin is scarred and splotchy but it is beautiful. My soul ached but is now healed. I was alone, and now I have you.

September 11 2016

It's still very hot here so Mom took Annie and Buddy to the lake yesterday to "test the waters." Annie loved it, Buddy not so much. However, I'm getting around well enough that Mom thinks I could get in with my Help Em Up Harness. So we will keep you posted. Annie and Buddy got baths in the yard when they got home. I slept on my left side again last night

Trip to lake: loved sniffing around. I swam but don't care much for it. I had a nice bath when I got home. Bella and Bucket are back. I spent a good while wobbling around back yard and have taken a special interest in the fat toad that waits on our back walkway every night. I don't do anything but sniff him enough to make him hop. Strange creature, all bumpy looking.

A special prayer to the victims who are still suffering from Sept. 11 fifteen years ago. To those who gave their lives, we will always remember you, to the families, our prayers for your hopes, and to ISIS and radical Islam, we won! We continue to win, and we always will.

September 13, 2016

We had a good time today, and I got to spend time in the yard several times because it is too hot.

So, Mom sings in the North Carolina Master Chorale, and she rehearses on Tuesday nights. Dad told her it was a solid four hours of us being jealous over who was getting attention and barking at the slightest noise. Odd how when she comes home, we are all quiet and settled in...of course, Mom baby talks to all of us and Dad doesn't, so that's a hint, Dad.

The original two of us were Annie and Bella as tiny puppies, then Bucket then Buddy and then Sandy. Oh and somewhere in between all of that came Lulu and Tipper. We own stock in lint rollers, and Mom says no pair of black pants will be allowed to leave the house without dog hair.

Please check your local shelters if you feel you could foster a homeless pet. You'd be sad at some of the reasons these poor babies were turned into shelters. And heartfelt thanks to our law enforcement officers who pull us out of ditches and out of the middle of highways, who notice when we are chained and in bad condition and get us to shelters. THEY ARE TRUE HEROES!!!

September 14, 2016

Some person in our house is going to a 45th high school reunion soon. We won't mention any names but since Mom and Dad are just two days apart in age, we will leave you guessing. We don't like suitcases that get brought out of some secret place and then get taken to the car, but we are lucky to have our good friends who will be staying with us!!!!!

I've been a happy girl today and woke up at my usual early time. It's a full-time job monitoring all these people (we call our canines and felines "people" too), and there is never a dull moment. Lulu has taken to sleeping in the bath tub in the master bath. We don't know why. Bella barks at anything that moves outside, Annie is just a sweetie, Buddy is a momma's boy, Bucket is a little love, and Tipper is the shy one. We are Mahoney's Menagerie!

I've been thinking that I'd make a really good president and all the others here could be my cabinet! I can monitor and watch and herd when necessary, Annie can be my secretary of state, Bella can be my secretary of defense, Buddy can be my secretary of welfare, Bucket can be my secretary of education, Tipper can be my secretary of the treasury, and Lulu can be secretary of the interior (of the bath tub). Sounds sane to us, compared to what is going on in the real insane election!!!!!

September 16, 2016

Mom is having a wonderful time and feels blessed to have grown up in a small town in the Blue Ridge Mountains in the Shenandoah Valley of Virginia!

Dad has met some of her classmates who had played ball when he did or lived in Florida or Saint Louis and was the husband extraordinaire!

I am home and all of us are loving being taken care of and spoiled!!!

Yes, Mom is the one who had the 45th reunion. It is a blessing to see so many friends with whom I grew up in a small industrial town where no one was a stranger. We didn't ever lock our back door, seldom our front door, never locked the car downtown, left the windows of the car rolled down, and never worried. Like so many of you, we played in the yard until way after dark in the summer. Our games were Kick the Can, King of the Mountain, Snipe Hunting, and more. September was always back-to-school month, and it was magic to begin to wear fall clothes and smell fireplaces burning. Classmates reunited who went from kindergarten to high school graduation together. There is no place like home.

September 19, 2016

Well, everyone is in their own beds, and Mom and Dad are all tuckered out from a weekend of reunion activities. We all got terribly spoiled while she was gone, but we really were glad to see them come home.

It's nice for me to be able to say there's no place like home!

Later this day:

This week marks 8 months of me really having a life. I've been in my new home for 8 months, and they originally told my mom and dad I would not live more than a few weeks. I am such a sweet happy girl that my family can't believe I could ever trust anyone after the abuse and neglect I suffered. One of the things I love to do every day is just stand in the yard and look around. I love sniffing the air and seeing the activity. I love to feel the rubs and hugs I get when my mom and dad get home so now I am always at the door with Annie and Buddy.

Please be careful of deer that are now on the roadside, and if you see one that has been killed, call the county you are in to come and dispose of it. We've seen numerous skunks, raccoons, and possums in the road lately who haven't survived the traffic. And if you see a neglected or abused animal, please don't just ride away or ignore it. Do the next right thing.

Yes, I am the one who stops in the middle of traffic to try to save the life of a poor scared dog or cat. I am the one who stops when a herd of deer is crossing. I am the one who will get out of the car and redirect traffic to go around a wounded animal. My husband often says that if he were lying in the yard with birds pecking at his eyes, and there was an injured animal just beyond him, I'd step over him to get to the animal. Not true, but it would cross my mind.

September 21, 2016

Dr. Ruth came today, and I had an acupuncture treatment thanks to my Go Fund Me account. We also found out we can get one of the prescription drugs much cheaper if we get a prescription from the vet instead of having them fill it. Mom and Dad are switching me over to a no-grain kibble because my canned food went up .20 a can. I really like the kibble and we are doing it slowly so my system doesn't get upset.

Mom found out there is a way to make a book of Facebook posts and is thinking of doing it. We really want to give back and maybe a book would inspire people to volunteer at shelters, to champion and support no-kill shelter laws, to give a home to a needy pup or cat. There's so much work to be done. Mom says if she was starting a career all over again, she would work for a shelter and raise awareness.

I want to show you what love and prayers and dedicated people have done for Augustus. He, too, is a miracle and another example of the difference you all make in one simple life. We all have but one life so let us live it well in the knowledge that every effort may one day save us all.

I wrote a post last night and somehow, it never showed up. I'm so sorry if you looked for one and I wasn't there.

Anyway, I am having a bit more trouble staying up on all 4 feet so Mom and Dad are thinking the three pounds I've gained may need to come off. Mom got the buzzy thing to trim Annie's nails and I immediately went to my "your bed" in the bedroom. I do not like that thing.

My new trick today was nosing the bedroom door until Mom opened it. Lulu is the one who goes around shutting doors, and while Mom was dressing this morning I decided I didn't like the door being shut … so I let Mom know I wanted in.

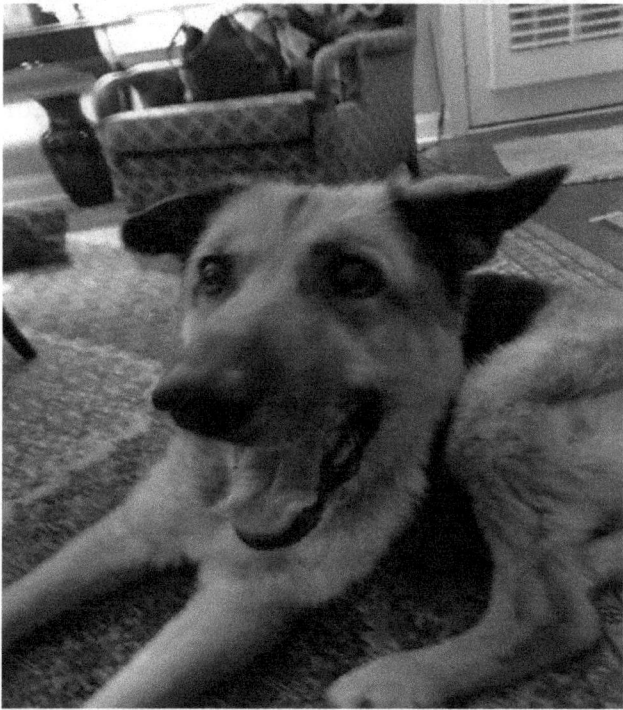

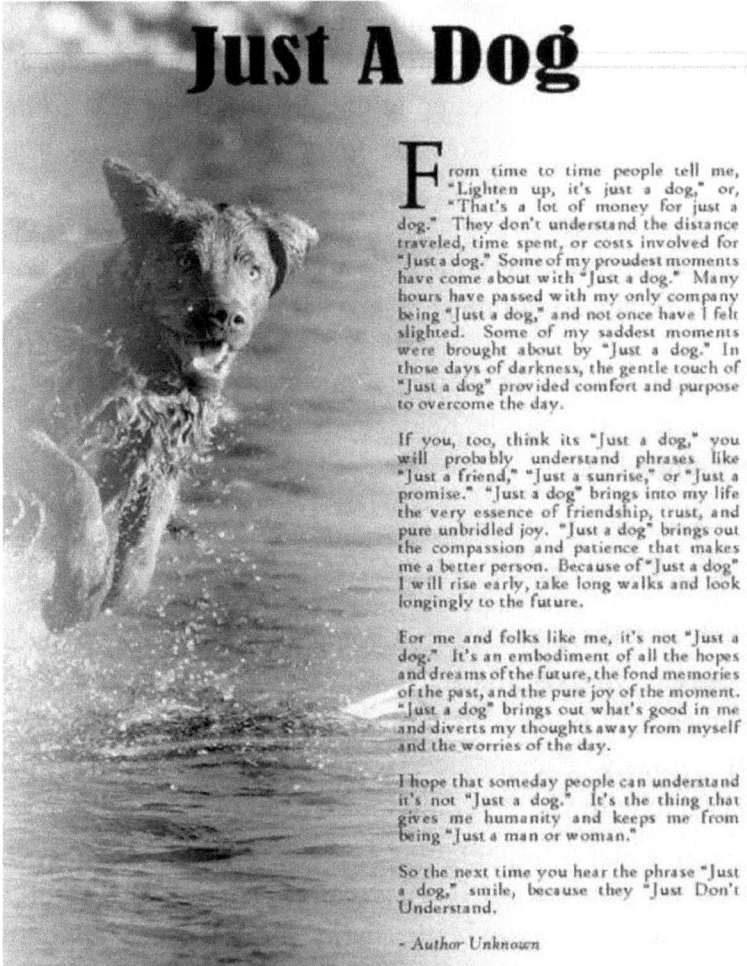

Just A Dog

From time to time people tell me, "Lighten up, it's just a dog," or, "That's a lot of money for just a dog." They don't understand the distance traveled, time spent, or costs involved for "Just a dog." Some of my proudest moments have come about with "Just a dog." Many hours have passed with my only company being "Just a dog," and not once have I felt slighted. Some of my saddest moments were brought about by "Just a dog." In those days of darkness, the gentle touch of "Just a dog" provided comfort and purpose to overcome the day.

If you, too, think its "Just a dog," you will probably understand phrases like "Just a friend," "Just a sunrise," or "Just a promise." "Just a dog" brings into my life the very essence of friendship, trust, and pure unbridled joy. "Just a dog" brings out the compassion and patience that makes me a better person. Because of "Just a dog" I will rise early, take long walks and look longingly to the future.

For me and folks like me, it's not "Just a dog." It's an embodiment of all the hopes and dreams of the future, the fond memories of the past, and the pure joy of the moment. "Just a dog" brings out what's good in me and diverts my thoughts away from myself and the worries of the day.

I hope that someday people can understand it's not "Just a dog." It's the thing that gives me humanity and keeps me from being "Just a man or woman."

So the next time you hear the phrase "Just a dog," smile, because they "Just Don't Understand."

- *Author Unknown*

September 24, 2016

(Just read the comments on tonight's post and found out a very lucky German Shepherd was rescued by a member of my Facebook family tonight!!!!! So excited and so very proud!)

I went on a walk tonight in my wheels. It's been weeks of temperatures in the 90s and then the monsoon this past week. Mom thought it was cool enough, so we went. I made friends through the fence with Chewy, my tiny little next-door neighbor Yorkie mix. I visited with some children and loved them. So tonight I am worn slap out. Mom put my rear feet up in the stirrups, and I was so fast down the walk that she had to slow me down.

Our hummingbirds have gone south and things are just beginning to wear themselves out with growing. Butterflies are far fewer than even a week ago so fall must be here. But today it was 91!

A prayer tonight for the rescuers who get calls any time of day or night and rush to help the neglected and abandoned, the lost and the hungry animals!!

September 26, 2016

THE BEST DEBATE EVER is going on between Bella and me. We are jockeying for position at Mom's feet ...I am using my shepherding techniques, and Bella is using her bully techniques. However, since I've previously campaigned for position, I am confident that shepherding will win over bullying! It's far more educational to watch how we negotiate and compromise and could possibly be something other people could learn from...we are now lying peacefully end to end. So much better than being snarky and growly. Mmmmmmm.

So tonight and tomorrow night, we all need to pray for our country.

September 28, 2016

My bath is tomorrow so that will wear me out. Had an ok day today. Some days are better than others. Mom and Dad will be headed out of town for a few days next week so we will be loved and taken care of by Lexi. Bella and Bucket will go home tomorrow so it will all be quiet here again. We are all ready for bed and want to remind you how much we love you and what a difference you have made in our lives. Mom and Dad could not have gotten me the treatments and the meds and the supplements without your kindness and support. We are all thankful that Buddy and Annie have stayed healthy during my recovery and therapy and praying everyone will continue to be ok for a while.

Huge thank you for your loyalty and your kind words to us because it really does help keep us going when the 5 a.m. wake-up call comes to go outside! Blessing on all of you and God grant us some good leadership to keep us strong and a nation of heroes.

September 29, 2016

Life got in the way today, and I didn't get my bath but will for sure in the next two days. I, for sure, am not as strong as I was last week but it may be due to the few pounds.... we are hoping. And we need to order more supplements because we haven't gotten a refill of the EFAC so maybe that's it. Mom and Dad have successfully cut down on the expensive canned food because it was crazy how expensive it was. We hope to continue the acupuncture sessions. It's $75 per session so we have to be mindful of costs of meds and therapy. I am, as it turns out, one expensive dog.

My mom says I am the most determined strong headed dog she's ever seen. But I so love children and all the animals I meet. If I'd had a good young life, I could have been a highly trained and skilled dog because I'm so smart. Sometimes it is hard to teach an old dog new tricks.

I understand "wait" and "ramp" and "potty" and "outside" and "bedtime" and "treat" and "daddy" and "Annie", "Buddy", "kitty", "water"... so, all in all, I'm doing pretty well for a dog who spent most of her life chained to a post.

If you live in the Raleigh or Triangle area, we want you to know about Dr. Ruth West, who comes to our home to help Sandy every two weeks, if possible on our part. Acupuncture has been so helpful, and Dr. West is so very good with her! She has given Sandy more time on 4 legs!

Yes, all of you have enabled my parents to provide the best of care for me. It has been a steady stream of veterinary treatments and therapy, but my mom and dad were determined that I should have a chance at a quality life after spending my years neglected and abused. Initially, I was to be euthanized after being confiscated from abuse. My namesake, Sandra, convinced a rescue to pull me and my rescue organization found my now mom and dad to foster me. I weighed around 58 pounds, had pus in my ears, had nails 4" long, completely covered in demodectic mange. I could not stand or walk and I wanted to die. My mom and dad reached out to all of you...... and I AM ALIVE! I can stand briefly on my own legs (I have severe spinal damage and DM) and can still walk about 5 steps before falling. Thanks to all of you, I am able to be on expensive meds, supplements, and excellent food. I have wheels that I love, I even have two of my very own beds.... one in our den and one in the bedroom. I have a family now too! I have a brother named Buddy, a sister named Annie, and two kitties named Lulu and Tipper. I have been treated at the North Carolina State Veterinary School and have therapy that has allowed me to occasionally be able to wag my tail. The light is back in my eyes, and although I know I'm old and it won't last forever, we are all grateful on a daily basis for my life and for all of the blessings bestowed on us by you.

Today is Sandy's human aunt's birthday. She is also a huge lover of animals and has had German Shepherds through the years. She has rescued and nursed back to health several and has welcomed them as members of her family.

October 1, 2016

At last, it was spa day!!!! I got the massage of a lifetime while lathered in warm water and shampoo!!! My legs, my tail, my tummy, my back, my neck and shoulders!!!! Then after being towel dried, I got the hairdryer on low to dry the places that stay damp because I lie down so much!! In addition, after dinner, we all got frozen marrow bones and I am now slap worn out. I am asleep on the rug with my head on my "your bed." A taste of the wonderful life! Blessings and gratitude!

October 2, 2016

Apparently, the massage and restarting the EFAC worked well. I slept all night on my LEFT side without being asked! And, I was a little steadier on my feet today! We revel in our miracles that happen every day. We are all so thankful.

Mom and Dad are so perplexed about this election thing. Truth, strength, courage, kindness, integrity... all so sadly missing. Dogs only see the truth...dogs show the best of courage and strength and love ...wonder what has happened to our humans.

We struggle to always find ways to relieve Sandy's pain and anxiety. Sometimes it is just hit or miss, and sometimes the arsenal of meds we have allows us to minimize her discomfort. Every moment of Sandy being pain free or even being more comfortable is a blessing.

October 5, 2016

No worries my Facebook friends. All is well here at home. Mom is just busy and took a break last night. Thinking so much of the victims of Matthew and the despair the people in Haiti and islands must feel. I know about despair and never want to have any dog or anyone have to go through it. So asking you tonight to say your prayers for them, because I know your prayers work!

October 7, 2016

We are not getting any bad weather except rain but keeping our hopes up that there will be no more loss of life with the floods and winds of Matthew. It's so easy these days to be pessimistic and disappointed in things that are going on in the world. My mom's favorite motto is "glass half full," so it is important that we count blessings. Life for me has been a mixed bag. Until 10 months ago, it was horrible and I know too well what it is like to be outside with no shelter and no food or anyone to care. I can't bear to think of the people who are in this situation because of mother nature. But, I am living proof that prayer and positive energies and healing wishes go a long way. So I'm counting on all of you, my Facebook Family, to send your healing thoughts and prayers to the victims and families of this terrible storm. My mom wants me to tell you that you all are the heroes in my life! She and my dad know this every day. I belong to every one of you, and know I am blessed by you.

October 8, 2016

We weren't predicted to have such a large amount of rain. But we got over six inches of rain, and North Carolina has massive flooding in many areas. If you have plans for visiting Raleigh or east of us, please check conditions before you travel.

We have been housebound all day but our house sits on a high elevation, so no flooding and only a few damaged trees.

Electricity was touch and go but we are fortunate that we have current.

So, if you live in an area that is unaffected and feel you could possibly go be a volunteer to help rescue animals, please contact your local shelter to find out how to help.

October 9, 2016

Since I am running for president, my mom is not supporting either of the two-legged candidates. She also does not like politics at all. So pardon the liberty she took. I made her take the previous post down. We are not a politically inclined family. We just believe in accountability and responsibility which is why I now have a home and food and you. Thanks for overlooking her rant.

Update on me: I had an upset tummy today and a bit of unpleasantness that came along with it. I got chicken and rice for dinner and will be getting it for the next few days. I didn't eat anything different or new so Mom figures it was from something I ate in the yard...... who knows?

It is a little chilly here after the big storm and I'm already feeling thankful for my cozy bed. Thankfully the sun was out today but the winds were really whooping around. I am still able to take myself to bed but need some assistance getting all of myself on the bed. Tomorrow am will be here in a few hours, so will say goodnight and sending prayers to flood victims and the scared animals.

October 10, 2016

Well, we are so blessed that we have electricity and no flooding. It is horrible here in many parts of North Carolina and we just got another flash flood warning. My house is in a high elevation and the creek is way below us, so we are not worried. I love this cool fall weather and it has made me rambunctious.

Many of our North Carolinians are in shelters and have lost everything from the flooding. Animal shelters are getting filled and rescue workers are even rescuing half-drowned deer and wildlife. Pray for them as they go about in the dark and as they fly helicopters to get to people.

October 13, 2016

Just some brief updates:

- My tummy is back to normal and I do love chicken and rice!
- Today was beautiful for us. It is devastating for so many just east of here.
- Dr. Ruth comes tomorrow!!!!!! I am so happy!
- Mom had rehearsal tonight so she is tired.

The treatments continue to be helpful, and Sandy truly gets excited to see Dr. Ruth. So many things have become available to us to help Sandy. It is just astonishing when I think of how many of you love her and read her story every night. By the way, when she really wants attention, she is very vocal and also finds a way to get to where she wants to go. Wobbly and stumbling, but she does it.

October 14, 2016

I got my acupuncture today, and big news! I had feeling in my feet and in the tip of my tail! Dr. Ruth was so pleased and I was frisky enough that she had to keep putting a couple of the needles back in because I was moving around trying to beg for another treat she brings with her!

I'm still very unstable on my feet and some days, I drag myself more than others. It's just the way it goes. So little is known about DM and there may be a chance that I only have severe spondylosis, which is sort of like stenosis in humans. But either way, I've got bad nerve damage in my hind end.

Will be letting you know if there is a foundation for spinal research on dogs...... could be a great resource.

I am one determined dog!! And my mom and dad have learned how smart I am. I have a new trick! I take things of my mom's from the bedroom to the den...... like socks and flip-flops...... Mom finally caught me in the act tonight with one of her slippers.

So thankful to be able to enjoy even the little things!

October 15, 2016

As we sit in our safe and warm and dry home tonight, we can't help but think of the thousands and thousands of people who will suffer from Hurricane Matthew. Hundreds of animals will also suffer and be without shelter. It is humbling to think of all we have and the abilities we have to prepare for disasters like this. Please send your best prayers and most positive energies to those who are and will suffer.

I am a happy, worn-out girl tonight. Annie gave up today and actually consented to play with me. I was so happy and wore myself out. Thought I'd tell you about a little trial my mom and dad did to see if there was a difference in me......so they took me off of the Gabapentin for a few days to see if there was a need to keep it up. Not noticeable the first day or second day but began to notice a slowing down the third day. So anyway after 5 days, I am back on it and much happier and active. I received the nicest card and gift from Michelle yesterday and appreciate all the devotion she has for me!! And, the curl in my tail is showing a little now! It was totally drooping and hanging down and now there's movement and a slight curl. Thank you for all the love and prayers for the flood victims. It's going to be a long, long recovery for them.

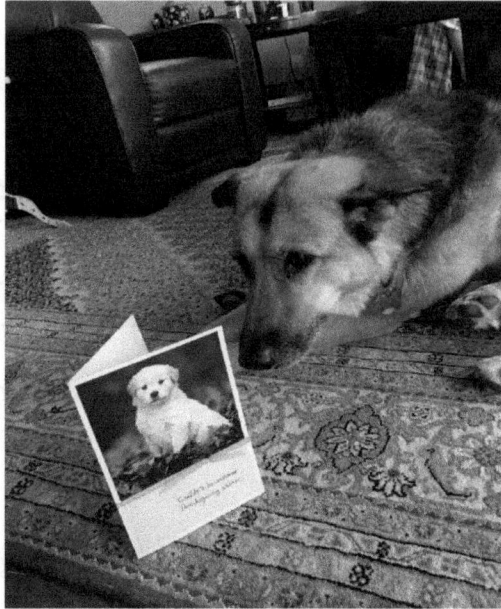

October 16, 2016

All is well with me and it was a fine day. Haha! Annie woke up before Me and started barking like a crazy dog! Some sound our neighbors made on an early morning to work .... anyway, she succeeded in waking the entire household.

We saw the saddest pictures today from the east coast towns of North Carolina. Some of the rivers crested and hundreds and thousands of people and businesses and roads are flooded. Most people lost everything, crops are ruined and the animal shelters are filled with every kind of animal you can think of. It is pitiful and when the water goes down, they will be left with muck and mud. Water systems are contaminated and places like Lumberton and Kingston and Goldsboro are begging for drinking water and toiletries and diapers, even underwear and socks and shoes. My mom has offered to meet people from her church in Richmond, where she used to live, when they come to North Carolina with donations to help distribute them.

If any of you my Facebook family can possibly foster a kitten or a chicken or a cat or a dog or a pup, please contact any of the animal shelters simply by looking them up on Google.

Parts of Interstate 95, the main north-south corridor of the USA are closed until November for flooding and repairs.

It's sad that the candidates who want votes can't even visit these areas to muster up support for these people who are suffering. I wish each of them would just take three minutes to acknowledge the anguish.

Thank you for your healing energies and surrounding love for me and my family.

October 17, 2016

My loving Facebook family: I have a special request tonight. One of our Facebook family friends has had a terrible day. Her baby Oscar was attacked by two other dogs and has a very long recovery ahead. Please send Oscar your prayers and your powerful healing energies because he needs all of it. I'm asking all my angels to surround him and his family with love and support and thoughts and prayers. I had a good day and am even looking for Dad or Mom when they go into another room! I've exercised my most pitiful whine and used my big voice at the shadows in the yard. I don't know why my mom thinks it's so amusing but she laughs when I bark! May you all rest well with peace in your dreams tonight and may your sleep be guarded by angels. And Oscar, you have no idea how powerful my Facebook family is. You will soon find out. Sending you our love!

October 18, 2016

Word reached us today of all the animal shelters in eastern North Carolina that are in desperate needs of supplies and help. Shelters are packed and there is no immediate relief in sight. Lumberton, Princeville, Kingston, and the list goes on. We will be packing up blankets and towels and extra leashes to send. I don't have the phone numbers but you can find the shelters by googling the flooded areas.

I was tired today; I guess I am usually tired the day after acupuncture but tonight I am fast asleep on my left side, giving my right side some relief. My right ear is a little foul so Mom has started the cleansing and antibiotic routine. I'm not terribly fond of it but tolerate it. Annie and Buddy and I love to get up at 6:00 a.m. to smell that fresh morning dew and whiff the first fragrances of the day. I am a blessed girl and your prayers have helped me so much in the past 8 months. I might even get something Mom calls a Christmas Stocking this year if I'm good. Buddy and Annie get excited when she asks them about theirs so I guess it's a good thing.

I'll keep you posted on those developments. Love to all of you always!

October 18, 2016

Blessings to all of you for sending Oscar so much love and so many prayers. I'll ask his mom for an update so I can pass it along to you. I slept on my left side the past two nights and am doing it again tonight. It seems to make me feel better to give my right side a rest. I have taken myself to bed before everyone for three nights in a row. Such a German Shepherd thing to do! My fur is worn a little thin from lying on my right side so much. My digestive system is fine now and I'm on a pretty steady diet of chicken and peas and rice. I've gotten to be pretty filled out compared to the 56 pounds I was.... no recent weight taken but you can tell by my pictures I have meat and muscle where I had none. I think I'll ask mom to take pictures of the steps I have to navigate to get to the yard and the ramps we have to make it easier for me. My GoFundMe account enabled Mom and Dad to get the ramps back a few months ago. It is really helpful. Thank you for every thoughtful thing you have passed along to Mom and Dad. Mom says we need to try every day to pay it forward, so tomorrow, do a kind deed.... take a cart from the parking lot into the grocery store with you and take it back in when you are done, pick up a piece of trash and throw it in a trash can, hold a door open, say hello in an elevator, thank the postman, thank a policeman...... these times need our kindness to others.

October 19, from Oscar

Well, it's been 24+ hours since those mean dogs attacked and tried to kill me. Mom keeps telling me how much she loves me and cries a lot. I'm still very sore but I want to get up and walk and even wagged my tail a few times today, especially when Dad came home from work. I go to see my doctor tomorrow and he'll make sure everything looks good and let Mom and Dad know how I'm healing. I mostly slept today and like it when Cabo is close to me. I ate some really good food and got up on my own to eat and drink. Thank you to everyone that has been thinking and praying for me.

October 21, 2016

I am a bit off today and Mom thinks I have an ear infection, so we will be calling the vet tomorrow morning. I've been very clingy to Dad and even nudged my way into the bathroom when he was showering. I don't like it when he leaves the house and I whine! Mom's working a lot lately and we are all hanging out being bored so tomorrow is "let's take a walk" day! My walks these days consist of going down the alley about 3 houses and walking to the boulevard a half block and back. After that I am exhausted. We all got up at 5:30 this morning ... Mom got up and tried to go back to bed but I wasn't having any of that! I wanted to be fed and wanted her in the room with me and Annie and Buddy. Mom's had a long day! I know my Facebook family is a group of loving kind people so it must be hard on all of you to see the USA in such an ugly political season. Prayers that hearts will open and kindness will win!

Here's the update on Oscar for today from Oscar himself:

Here's Day 3, thanks for sharing!! Hugs and kisses to Sandy! Well it's day 3, and other than not being able to poop, I'm doing ok. I seem a little skittish but Mom says that's to be expected given that those big dogs were so vicious. My bruising and swelling is looking yucky but Mom says hopefully that's because it's healing. All my wounds that are stitched up look good. I went to work with Dad today and I liked seeing everyone that comes in, but I'm pretty tired tonight. Mom said she's tired too, and we'll be going to bed soon. As always, thanks for keeping me in your thoughts and prayers. Love, Oscar

October 22, 2016

I did get a trip to the vet today. They are so good to me!!! Got my nails trimmed and medicine for my ear infection. I have been low-key because going to the vet is still stressful for me. Mom and Dad both went with me and Dad tried to wait out in the waiting room. I was having none of that so he had to come in the examining room too. The doctors think I'm pretty incredible and are so interested in the supplements I take and how they make a difference. Methyl B12 and turmeric are wonderful!! It is getting to really be fall here, so Mom says, and I love sniffing the cool air. Who knew I'd ever live to see another fall? I know I talk a lot about how your love and prayers work, but every breath I take and every step I take are a pure miracle. The healing light and warmth from your energies has made this life I have possible. Each one of you should know how very important you are to me and that my family offers prayers of thanks for you every day. You all being part of my life has made a huge difference to me and to my family. They never set out to be heroes and could not have come this far without you all. Please know each of you is loved by us.

October 23, 2016

Mom sang a concert today ... Handel's Alexander's Feast. So Dad and us kids watched football. Tomorrow may be a nice crisp day for a walk.

I've had to go back on chicken and rice...tummy upset again. We don't know why but my mom and dad will figure it out. I got praised for being such a good girl and asking to go out as soon as I needed to. I do this by walking up to either Mom or Dad and just staring at them. They know!

Rest with peace and sleep deeply, dear friends

October 24, 2016

I am a sick pup today. My intestinal problems worsened overnight and Dad was up twice and Mom once to take me out. I'm so drained and mom's trying to make sure I drink water. Vet found out I have a significant bacterial infection so I'm on antibiotics as well as probiotics to try to get my system balanced. I did eat my breakfast and dinner (chicken and rice) and just plain don't feel good. Tomorrow will be better! I know many of you fight each day to feel better and to heal and beat the odds. Please know you all are in my family's prayers.

It's not fun having tummy problems and today it continued so I am on a rice and chicken diet for a while with no dog food...... I have been really good about letting Mom and Dad know when I must go outside so tonight could be up and down for all of us. If it's not markedly better by morning, Mom will take the required sample to the vet to see what they think is going on. Annie and Buddy went for a walk but I'm really wrung out so I didn't go. Maybe tomorrow.

The east coast of North Carolina is just now shoveling mud out of the homes that were underwater and people are hoping to return home this week from the shelters. Some don't know if they have anything left. The animal shelters all over eastern Carolinas are overwhelmed so please share my post in case there is anyone willing to foster or who would adopt a dog or cat in need.

Thank you!!!

October 26, 2016

Well, the jury is still out on if I am better. I am on antibiotics and probiotics...... and now my intestinal troubles have caused me to have to eat pumpkin purée... and if that doesn't work in two days, it's back to doctor for me. We are so thankful for your prayers and loving wishes for me to feel better. I am drinking water and eating with a good appetite; just hoping it moves along, if you know what I mean.

Mom got in late last night because of rehearsal but we got up at 6 this morning. Mom went to the Highpoint Market for the day so she's pretty whipped. I am lying on my left side (yay!) and off to a deep sleep.

Today is a prayer for our country.... such hatred being spread, pitting American against American. Such a terrible election campaign..... Mom keeps saying she just wants it to be over and that she doesn't know what the country has come to. Isn't it a sad comparison when you compare the electoral candidates to the champion baseball teams...... such degradation between candidates and rampant yellow journalism versus sportsmanship and unity of fans in a match-up that everyone loves and respects. Here I go again campaigning.

October 28, 2016

Feast or famine around here today. Made quite a few trips to the yard and as the day progressed, things got more normal. I am eating and taking my medicine so tomorrow will be better.

We are keeping Bella and Bucket so it's the five of us for the weekend. Lulu ignores them but Tipper runs, which makes Bella want to chase her, so Mom had to fuss at her twice.

Mom and Dad have decided that they won't be handing out candy at Halloween because it is a bit unnerving to me to have the doorbell ring and I try to run to the door but just can't. Our house will be dark, and we will be spending money on acupuncture for me and not for 20 bags of candy.

It's going to be a warm, beautiful weekend. I'll be able to take a walk tomorrow.

And so tonight, please pray for the week to be strong and the fearful to have comfort and the starving and abused to be loved.

October 31, 2016

Happy Halloween to all my FB family. My day was good but wobbly, and we are still hopeful the back legs will line up again. Being sick really took me downhill. We are hoping to swing a visit for acupuncture this week.

Can't believe it's November! I never thought I'd see another one, and this Thanksgiving I'll be especially thankful for my "your bed," my blankets, my toys, my brother Buddy and sister Annie and for my kitties Tipper and Lulu. I'm feeling secure and loved and happy. What a life change!

Bella and Bucket's mom came to dinner tonight and to have some mom-and-dad time. The day here was beautiful and I did the normal routine of awaking at 6:30, getting help to go out, then breakfast, then once mom was sufficiently wide awake, I went back to sleep. These very warm October days have delayed all the trimming of shrubs and rose bushes and even the patio furniture is still in place. I am not complaining because I got to enjoy some time outside!

I am still on antibiotics and on the stuff for my ear. Our kitchen counter continues to look like a pharmacy. Mom says she is going to get me a pill box so she can get all this stuff off of the counter. Pretty good idea!

Happy All Saints to all of you! Seems all this Halloween stuff has taken over the true All Hallows Eve, a Christian tradition. Leave it to a GSD to know that. Anyway, no tricks around here but we do get treats quite often.

It is so interesting to see how All Saint's celebrations in the Roman Catholic and protestant religions are so different and reverent versus the spooky and garish holiday we call Halloween. I think dogs probably prefer All Saints Sundays to the persistent doorbell or the high-pitched excitement of children who trick or treat.

Eve of All Saints Prayer

Father,

All-Powerful and Ever-Living God,

Today we rejoice

in the holy men and women

of every time and place

May their prayers

bring us your forgiveness and love

We ask this through Christ our Lord. Amen.

From the Liturgy of the Hours

November 1, 2016

I was such a good girl this morning! I slept until 7:45 and so did Buddy and Annie! By the end of the day, I am one tired girl!

So mom has figured out that the new bottle of Dasaquin does not have the MSM in it that the previous bottle did. Horses have been getting MSM for years and now it is in glucosamine for us and humans. We don't know if that is making the difference but we will be getting the one with MSM ASAP!

Thank you for all the well wishes! I am working on it!!

Mom's work entered a contest for the best display window in Lafayette Village. So, today all of my two-legged sister's old stuffed animals came out of the attic. Mom's doing a forest with a doghouse and all the kitties and doggies from the attic and a life-size little girl doll with a red velvet dress, and if we win, all the award money goes to Second Chance Animal Shelter here in Raleigh. So if you happen to shop in Lafayette Village later in November, vote for Watkins Flowers of Distinction to win! I will post pictures after she gets it done!

What a stroll down memory lane it was getting all those much-loved stuffed animals out of the attic. My daughter loves animals and has three dogs and a horse. That apple didn't fall very far from the tree! Some treasures found too. The old Miller and Rhodes Christmas Bears and the Leggie Bears from Leggett Department Stores all carefully packed away. Even found the Cat in the Hat and the Grinch.

November 2, 2016

Special request! My human sister, who is 29, must have surgery on her back tomorrow. She has bad discs in L4 and L5. Would you please say a prayer for her that angels hold her hand while she is asleep and that the blessing of skilled hands be guided by God. Mom is pretty preoccupied with this right now.

By the way, thanks to help from my Facebook Family, I had acupuncture today from Dr. Ruth. I'm up and around and seem to be a bit better today!! I love me some Dr. Ruth.

November 2 (evening):

All is well. Mom is with my big sister and Dad is home with us. Many many thanks for all the prayers for her and us!

November 3, 2016

Who invented this Daylight Savings Time thing when you spring forward and fall back? Who thought that was a good idea? Talk about a body's 24-hour clock! I am all over it, and so are Buddy and Annie. Dad thought he'd take a tiny nap at 5 which was 6 to us and I had to body slam the bed to make sure he knew it was NOT ok with me to wait until 7:00 DST, 6:00 EST to eat!!! Now if you are confused, just think how we feel. So since I think it's 10:00 pm, I'll be taking myself to bed here in a minute. Mom and I had a nice leisurely tour of the backyard today and I loved the slightly crisp air and no bugs! Mom and Dad stored all the patio stuff today and took in plants because we are supposed to have frost tonight. I found one of my tennis balls in the process. Tonight we are hoping and praying for a united United States, for healing of hearts and minds, for redirecting turmoil to peace and goodness. After all, I know that prayers work!!! Just look at me! So saddle up and take the high road. Feed the hungry, nourish the sick, teach others to fish, lead by example, pay it forward, and treasure this life all the way into home plate!

Running in so many directions and not focusing on one direction at a time is my nemesis. Good thing I have a wonderfully focused better half and a GSD that keeps track of every move I make. Sandy is pretty vocal if she thinks it's time to eat or time to get attention. I may be scattered at times, but these fur babies keep me grounded. I have the common "why did I come into this room" moments, can't find my glasses moments, and go to another task before I am finished the current one. Sound familiar?

November 9, 2016

The sun did come up this morning and now Mom says it's up to each one of us to do right and teach right and live right. And crown thy good with brotherhood from sea to shining sea!

My dad had a fall off of his bike and now has a broken collar bone, and surgery scheduled for next Wednesday. He will need a plate and bone graft, so we are all dependent on mom for quite a while to come. She says for someone who is supposed to be retired she sure is tired!

I'm doing ok, and Mom is trying to teach me to eat out of a standing bowl. I am used to being fed with a fork, because I hate putting my nose into my food and because I am spoiled. Mom says I need to learn because she's taking care of Dad and working part-time and singing and taking care of my human sister. I did ok tonight and ate half of my food on my own. Mom says I'm such a big girl and that I'm beautiful. I'm very much a schedule type of dog who likes everything to happen at the same time of day every day, so I'm still waking at 6:30 daylight savings time which is 5:30 Eastern Standard Time. Mom's on full-time escorting me to the yard duty so she is thinking Christmas decor this year will be very minimal and she is a Christmas maximalist!

Dad is lucky to have a great doctor at Duke Orthopedic!

November 10 2016

So Dad was at home being still, and Mom was at work. Sister is doing better and Mom will be home all day tomorrow! Yay!

Dad watched a lot of news today. It seems there are a lot of humans at odds with each other over something called "politics" and "elections". I've been hated and called names in my previous life. I'm guessing the hateful people in this world and the people who want to make life harder by disagreeing and using violence are really missing the joy of being alive, of being free, of having food, and of having a place to sleep ...and a place to learn...I would have had joy all my life if I'd had those things. But I have joy now.

November 12, 2016

I was restless today. And ate like a horse. Mom massaged my hind legs and I am better now.

Thank you to all of my Facebook Family for keeping me and my family in your hearts. My life is not very adventurous, but I am so happy and just love sharing with all of you. My hind legs are a little less useful these days but I am still able to stand and that is a huge accomplishment. I walk two or three steps and Mom has yoga mats all over the kitchen and den and master bedroom so I can manage.

As cold weather sets in I think about the neglected and abused and homeless dogs and kitties. We always pray that one day it will change.

November 14 2016

This won't be long tonight because Mom is tired and so am I but had to tell you what I did today. It was a beautiful high 60s outdoors and I went out with Mom. She decided to let me maneuver on my own and I had such a nice, wobbly time. I smelled the ground where the tomato plants had been and sniffed every tree and bush in the backyard! I laid in the yard and watched mom sit on the steps. It was a good 30 minutes and it made me tired but happy.

It's the little things, isn't it, that are so wonderful to be able to do. Sleep well, my friends!

November 15, 2016

It was a busy busy day. Mom was a whirling dervish with cutting rose bushes back and laundry and grocery store and rehearsal, and Dad's surgery on his collar bone is tomorrow.

I enjoyed the backyard for a while and was pretty insistent about my dinner. We got a lovely Thanksgiving card and mom took pictures of me reading it! It's hard to believe It's already the middle of November.

Mom's work is sponsoring a rescue organization in their display window. If the window wins the prize for the best in the shopping village, then the rescue gets a prize plus a dollar for every vote that is cast. Mom decorated the window with stuffed animals that were my sister's. Puppies and kitties and bunnies and even a swan on a lake in front of a forest.

So if you are in wondering what to give someone for Christmas, pick your local shelter and make a donation of any size in that person's honor. That's how I found my forever home! My mom and dad gave a Christmas gift in honor of someone who loves German Shepherds, and the rescue called my mom when they were in desperate need of a foster. Mom and Dad said yes!!!!

November 16, 2016

All went well with Dad. Thanks to all my FB family for thoughts and such healing wishes! Mom's on nurse duty every two hours so post is brief tonight. I was such a good girl and didn't make a bit of mess the whole day while they were gone to outpatient from noon until this evening! Mom was very very proud and thankful!

November 17, 2016

We are all doing well...Mom has to get up every two hours so posting will be a little lean the next couple of days.

Love and blessings to all. Thanks from Dad for all the kind wishes and prayers! I write the posts, Mom interprets, and Mom types them on her phone. Sometimes, Mom gets so busy interpreting that she gets fat fingers and words look funny.

November 18, 2016

I'm fine and just want to say good nite and sleep well!

November 21, 2016

We all just want to take a minute to wish my Facebook Family a wonderful Thanksgiving and an enjoyable weekend. Our blessings are abundant and we know your prayers and the healing energies you have sent me are the reason I am able to celebrate my first Thanksgiving with a happy heart, a warm home, a nice "your bed," great food and the love of a family. We never forget that our Facebook family has made this life possible, and as a special Thanksgiving treat, I had a visit from Dr. Ruth today and had a wonderful acupuncture session. We will be celebrating with family and are thankful for all the things we so often take for granted: fresh air (thinking of those fur babies in the forest fires), warmth, food, friendship, freedom (yes, we are free !!!!), and for all the tireless efforts of the many rescue organizations who are determined to save us all! They are working as you read this, so stop for just a moment and ask angels to wrap them in courage and strength. Spread the thankfulness and count the blessings.

November 23, 2016

Saving Sandy updated their status.

Back to the doctor for Dad today. He will be in the sling for at least three more weeks. Then Mom's day was filled with something called an "oil change" which makes no sense to me. I had a good day outside several times and now we are falling into our beds.

Thinking about all the reasons to be thankful.

She is so funny. She follows our every move, and her eyes plead for us not to go out of the door. She would be such a Velcro dog if she could get around. This sweet soul asks for nothing and is so grateful for just being loved.

November 26, 2016

All the leftovers were eaten tonight but not by me because I don't get people food. I get a special diet so my tummy doesn't get upset, but I get plenty! I'm so excited to have my first Christmas!!! All the lights and smells are different around the house and Mom is busy climbing the ladder and putting sparkly things out! Buddy and Annie and I are all curled up in the den while Dad watches......FOOTBALL AND MORE FOOTBALL!

I am still able to wobble a bit outside by myself and I am still walking, although wobbly, to my "your bed" in the bedroom and to my water dish. My dad and mom are very proud of me that I still let them know when I need to go outside 95% of the time. Sometimes when I'm in a deep sleep, I wet my bed but not frequently. I still take all my meds and supplements and believe me, MSM in my Dasaquin makes a difference!

Last Christmas, I was outside starving and covered with mange. This Christmas, my mom says I'll even get a stocking!

I hope your Thanksgiving was peaceful and that the day was kind to you. We are lucky to have family (yes, my human sis is doing well with her back.... slow but sure), and I know so many dogs and many of you might not be as lucky as we are. Please know we said a special Thanksgiving prayer for each of you! You all are high on our list of things for which we are thankful. (But I'm still wishing I had gotten some of the gravy!)

We received a wonderful recording of Sandy's Polka from our friend, and are so blessed to have friends who love us!!

The energy of the Season is all around us and we are happy to be sharing these days with you!

Comments from me during this holiday season may be few and far between. I always seem to bite off more than I can chew, and I've got quite a mouthful this year. Of course, if I would just not decorate every square inch of the house, it might be less hectic. Oh, how I love Christmas and the season and the sparkles and the lights. Christmas music fills my house and my car!

<u>November 27, 2016</u>

The glitter is everywhere! Mom keeps running that noisy thing over the floors and there is sparkly stuff shedding more than I do. By the way, I do like being brushed very much, but every time the brush comes out, so does Tipper, the short-haired kitty. Looks like she could find some other time to want to be brushed. I enjoyed some outdoor time today and remember that this time last year I was cold and had no fur and little to no coat. Miracles do happen, and I am one of them.

I got a note from one of my Facebook friends about adopting from a German Shepherd rescue. Most rescues can't afford to check out a potential home for a dog or cat if it is far away. Checking out the adopting parent is a big part of their process to make sure we adopted ones go to a good home that will meet our very own needs. But most every state has a German Shepherd Rescue and many have rescue places that shelter all kinds of dogs. Here the ones I know about are

Second Chance Animal Rescue and Shelter and we have Saving Grace, and Southeast German Shepherd Rescue.

Please remember that your Shelter needs all your old towels and blankets and dog beds and kitty beds. They rely on all these donated supplies to keep the babies waiting to be adopted warm. So instead of wondering what to do with those things, drop them off at the nearest shelter. A cold homeless baby will so appreciate it.

Here's Annie watching over me

To find rescues in your area, you can simply search online, and most of them at least have a phone number. Most breeds have shelters that are largely breed and mixed breed facilities. If they don't ask for a home interview or a lengthy interview on the phone, they really are not looking out for the welfare of the animals. Adopt, don't shop!

November 28, 2016

It was a long busy day yesterday so I didn't get to post. Too many things going on. These two weeks are Mom's busiest in the year. She has rehearsals every night and three concerts this weekend to sing and three next week. Dad is feeling a bit lonely in the evening. He goes back to surgeon today and hopes he can come out of the sling.

Thus begins the season of glitter. Glitter in my hair, on my face, on my clothes, in my pores. It goes down into the rugs and won't all come out until sometime mid-spring at the umpteenth vacuuming. I love it. The more sparkle, the better.

November 29, 2016

It was an early morning for me and by 8:30, Mom had done 4 loads of laundry. I had a good day because of all the messages I received about people doing things to help animals this Christmas and to raise awareness of how many homeless there are!

Buddy has some way hurt his left shoulder or left front paw and is hopping around on three legs, so he is off to vet in the morning with Mom.

We are all beat, so more from us tomorrow. Thanks to all of you for helping your local animal shelters!!!

November 30, 2016

I am just completely without words to thank each of you for your contributions to my GoFundMe page. It is a blessing, a miracle, an inspiration. We are so blessed with the love and care of our Facebook Family.

December 1, 2016

I had to go in the big glass box yesterday for a bath. It completely wore me out, but I had enough hair come off that we could have made a miniature German Shepherd.

My latest trick was going to the potty on the back sidewalk instead of on the grass. Mom wasn't pleased.

So today begins, and I hope it is a good experience for all things bright and beautiful!

Hi to all my FB family. Several of you have asked if I have a wish list on Amazon. I do and it is available if you go to Amazon and search for Saving Sandy. The items that I normally use for meds or baths are there or pads that Mom uses to protect my "your bed." But there is a kind of bed listed that is waterproof and might eliminate the need for pads because it can be washed. Anyway, you will need to go to shopping list page and search from there. Thank you for wanting the list. Please know all of you are always with me and your encouragement helps my mom and dad so so much. Mom thinks about all of you in the early early morning when she's half asleep taking me out to the yard and reminds herself how blessed we all are because of you.

December 2, 2016

Here are some things I heard Mom say today:

"These Christmas ornaments multiply while they are stored in the attic."

"Why did I come in this room?"

"I don't know what I've done with my glasses."

"The tree looks like it's leaning forward to me."

"No, I'm going to finish this before I start anything else."

"What in the name?"

"Why does that candle keep coming on in the afternoon?"

"If I'd put my shoes away, I wouldn't keep tripping on them."

"This ladder has got to go. It's in my way."

"Why is it so hot in here?"

"Oh my gosh this ceiling fan is filthy."

"The next house I have is going to have a Christmas tree closet where you just roll the tree in and leave it decorated."

"I'm just going to leave this stuff up all year."

She talks to herself a lot......

But I got to be outside for 45 minutes today! Mom and Dad were talking to neighbors, and I wandered around the backyard! It was wonderful!

I'm so excited about all these lights and sparkly things and there's a tree growing in our den! Our house smells like some kind of tree, and there are all these little elf people looking at me wherever I go. There's a little man beside the fireplace with a long white beard. He's sort of fat and has a bag of toys over his shoulder. He doesn't ever say a word. He just stands there. He's not nearly as tall as my dad and he's a lot older too. This Christmas thing is looking like it's something pretty special. I'll keep you posted about the little man beside the fireplace.

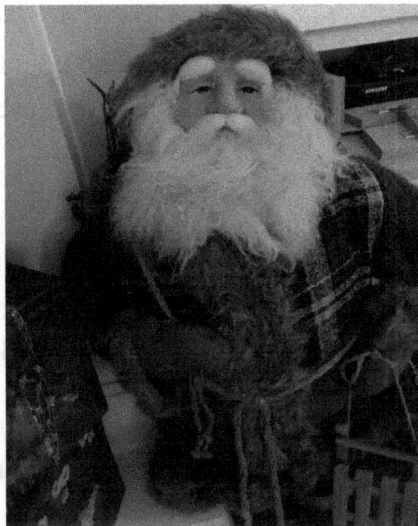

December 3, 2016

Well, he didn't move! He didn't move all day so I think he's trying to convince me he's doing things while I'm sleeping. He just stands there with his hand on his hip like he knows something I don't. Mom and Dad were gone much of the day, busy with concerts and doctor appointments. We were all very good babies while they were gone so we got extra treats tonight!

The jury is still out whether Buddy and Annie know what's up with the man beside the fireplace. Buddy is never very talkative but Annie cuts a wide swath when walking close to him, but she's not sayin' just yet. And now, on our piano are these tiny people. There is a shepherd and three guys who look like kings. And there's a donkey and a man and woman with a tiny baby lying on something that looks like hay. Oh, and there are angels everywhere in that room. Small ones, but I know about angels because of all of you!

December 4, 2016

He moved! I didn't see him, but he's not in the same spot. I was extra careful today to nap in the bedroom so he couldn't watch me. But I think he must have crept in and gone back because he's not in the same spot!

One of my Facebook friends suggested I get my mom to post all my expenses per month. So after she reviews all the receipts, she says she will ...... my friend wants us to do this because she believes all my friends and anyone who rescues a special needs dog needs to know.

So tonight, I'm thankful for treats and sparkling lights and for the clean yard Mom keeps every day! It makes going outside so much more pleasant! She says as soon as Dad's shoulder heals that he'll be back on poop patrol.

December 5, 2016

I got Mom up early this morning just to make sure that old man by the fireplace was still in the same spot. He was, so after I went out, I let Mom go back to sleep for a little while.

Mom keeps bringing these big boxes out of the attic, and now there's another little man sitting in a sleigh. I wonder where all these things were that are coming out of that place called the attic. Today, there was an incident of thievery when someone took treats out of the pantry when Mom and Dad went to Lowes. The usual suspect is Annie. But someone got into the pantry and got chews.

My eyes are slamming shut.

December 6 2016

I saw my mom move the bearded man when she vacuumed. Other than that, I don't think he has even blinked and I don't have any idea when he gets any sleep. Of course he may see me when I am sleeping. So for folks who rescue and foster disabled dogs, this list will be no news but since so many of you have helped me live another year (as of this coming January), I thought I'd respond to my Facebook friend who asked about my expenses.

Here is what I take: Rimadyl 2x/day, Tramadol 2x/day, Gabapentin 2x/day, Methyl Vitamin B12 2x/day, Turmeric 1x/day, EFAC 2x/day Dasaquin with MSM 2x/day. My annual senior comprehensive exam: $509 once per year. My Average monthly vet bill: $128. My acupuncture 2x/month: $150 Rimadyl: $87.00/month Gabapentin: $16/month Tramadol: $33/ month Dasaquin: $86/3 months Malaseb: $38/ 2 months Pee pads: $22/ Florazil: $13/mo Food: $64/mo

So isn't it just amazing how well I am doing! Anyway, thanks and love to many friends who have constantly said prayers for me and have kept me on my feet. Mom and Dad say how thankful they are because it really has taken a village to keep me alive!

I am a happy girl and extremely jealous of all the others that live with me! I have no trouble with whining and letting them know I want attention more than anyone else gets! I am soooo excited about Christmas and love all the activity! Sparkles are everywhere, and Mom and Dad seem to be in particularly good spirits.

NOTE: In editing this book, I have intentionally included the pricing of items that benefitted Sandy with arthritis and failing limbs. Awareness and education are so important in rescuing a compromised animal, and without the support of our Facebook family, we would not have been able to provide as we did for her.

December 7, 2016

I started early today, and I let Mom get a cat nap in after I had breakfast. Once the inside is completely decorated, Mom will TRY to take a photo of all of us in front of the fireplace. (Herding cats is problematic!) Mom and Dad spent most of the day outside, and I couldn't figure out what they were doing. Turns out there are a whole lot of new lights outside!

Please remember that your local shelters need blankets, towels, sheets, dog food, and cat food, and welcome your help! We have our car loaded with old blankets and towels and some dog food I would not eat. Here's the official lighting of the Mahoney house.

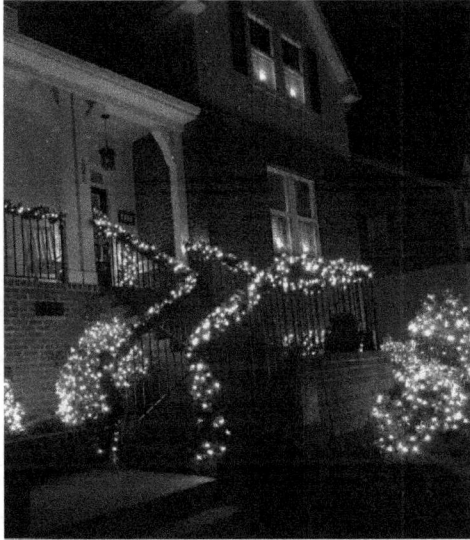

December 8 2016

That man beside the fireplace has a name. He is called Santa......which Mom says means "saint". I just can't figure out what a saint is and what he's doing in our house.

Mom says he's here to watch over us, but I think he's here to spy on me!

I have a habit of whining in the evening before bed. I've been doing this for a long time, and Mom worries. Dad says he doesn't know what I want. They walk around trying to retrieve my toy or seeing if I have water. Tonight they might have caught on that I whine when Annie or Buddy gets too close to Dad if he's eating something or if I just want to be possessive. Uh oh!

And it looks like winter weather is going to be around for a while now. It's very cold outside and I'm wearing my wonderful coats again!

We also follow Trio Animal Foundation Facebook page, and we are so happy tonight that Halo has found her forever home! She is such an inspiration and makes my heart proud of us survivors!

Again, none of us would survive without rescue organizations and foster families, and we hope you will share our stories to help the entire world understand more about animal abuse. Mom says most of the wisdom she has, if any, has come from loving an animal.

December 9 2016

Brrrrrrr! I don't know what happened between Wednesday and today but it is freezing cold, and I am not strolling in the night air now! I'm so thankful for my warm coats and warm home.

I know I thank you all the time for your kindness and your prayers. It seems like just words sometimes but I would not be alive to see Christmas or to experience the change of seasons, to feel the pats on my head and have my tummy full, to wobble to the side of the bed to tell Mom or Dad it's morning and I need to go out. None of this is without the miracles of love that have surrounded me during the past year. It was one year ago that I was confiscated/taken to a high-kill shelter. I had given birth to multiple litters and been left to starve and freeze and die. I spent last Christmas in the shelter as the clock ticked down towards the day of my euthanasia. Southeast German Shepherd Rescue and a woman named Sandra were determined to find me a foster home. And I waited...

December 10, 2016

It was a crazy night and morning. Mom and Dad stayed up to watch a tiny little girl so her mom could go have fun with my human sister. They went to bed at 3:00 this morning. Of course that didn't matter to me, so I got up at my usual 6:00 ...... and since I don't like them to go back to bed after I get up, I didn't let them get much rest. Mom ran that machine that makes a lot of noise all over the house today. She did things in a backwards order because then she brushed all of us and had to do the machine again. She talked to herself a lot about that.

Tipper and Lulu seem to think Mom put the tree up just for them and they promptly curled up on the thing that goes around the bottom of the tree. They didn't leave room for any of us either!

I have new boots!!!! They come up the bottom of my leg and will stay on so my feet don't get frostbitten or wet. I DO NOT LIKE WET FEET!

So this week, Mom says she's going to bake, and somewhere in that plan are homemade dog treats. She has two concerts this coming week so we will see how she makes time to "bake".

Our prayers tonight are for each of you to know you are loved, that you matter, and that you have many blessings.

December 11, 2016

Today: 9:00 am

Mom (still half asleep): "Good morning. Wow, it's 9:00!"

Dad: "Yes it's 9:00. What are you doing up so early?"

Mom: "I didn't even hear the dogs."

Dad: "I got up as soon as this one (pointing to Annie) started making all the noise, and that one (pointing to me) started body-slamming the bed."

Mom: "Thanks for getting up. I was really tired. Plus I was having an awful dream."

Dad: "About what?"

Mom: (standing by coffee maker) "I don't know. I can't remember."

Me: (thinking to myself) How does she walk from the bedroom to the den to the kitchen in less than one minute and forget what she was dreaming but remembers it was awful?

So the candles are all aglow in the windows and Mom is super excited about finding out how to upload all her wonderful Christmas CDs to her IPad. Boxing and labeling starts tomorrow she says. I'm now going to sleep on my left side!!!! Yay.

December 13, 2016

It was another day of having a bit of an upset stomach but Mom and Dad got right on it with chicken and rice and probiotics. Right now, I'm enjoying lying here with my dad and I am one thankful dog.

Mom and Dad got home late last night after the Christmas concert by the North Carolina Master Chorale. Mom sings in the chorale and Dad went to hear the concert. Both of them were whooped but not too tired to walk us and give us our bedtime treats. Mom has one more concert to sing with the Master Chorale Chamber Choir tomorrow night in Chapel Hill.

I think I've told you about Buddy taking all the toys into the dining room where he thinks we can't get to them. So tonight was the weekly round-up and I reclaimed several of the toys. I was in the process of trying to unwrap one of the presents under the tree that is NOT for me so Mom went and got an armful of my toys from the dining room. I guess I got her attention!

Remember that if you shop on Amazon, go to Amazon Smile and shop from there. It's the same Amazon, but by shopping on the smile page, part of your purchase can go to a charity of your choice. Many shelters are helped this way.

December 14, 2016

Oops. Mom fell asleep after rehearsal last night, and I couldn't wake her.

December 16, 2016

I'm back! I had to take a little break last night because Mom wasn't around to help me spell. She sang in her last concert of the season in Chapel Hill last night.

And... it seems that the man beside the fireplace with the white hair on his face is here for a reason. I've determined that it is indeed a special time of year because under that tree that is covered with shiny twinkling things are boxes wrapped in paper. And I LOVE to chew up paper. Mom thinks it probably is because I had to scrounge for food in trash before I was rescued. She didn't get mad but she and Dad moved all the boxes to where I can't see them. NO FUN! The man beside the fireplace must have told on me.

My tummy is back to normal and Dad is out of his sling. Mom is very glad about both. My dad asked Mom today if she had been inviting neighborhood dogs to use our yard. Ha! That because Mom didn't get around to poop patrol yesterday.

I am loving wearing my coats because it is really cold here now. And I have a new dog mat that goes just inside the back door. It keeps me from slipping and dries my feet off at the same time. Now that is really a double duty rug!

I am feeling so very lucky to be in a warm cozy home. I am so lucky to have so many Facebook friends. Christmas time can be so lonely for so many people and it is hard to be without people and fur babies we love. But all of us want you to know we will be here and all of you will be in our hearts. Your comments and good wishes are read and loved by us. It's because of your prayers and goodwill that I am still able to stand and wobble. They said I would decline so much more than I have. I am proof of being loved and of the power we have to help each other!

December 17, 2016

I've decided I really like the fireplace. It is so warm and makes me want to lie down and stretch out. Mom learned a new trick tonight. She read that dogs who have spinal issues and are down in the back end will often whine at night. It seems some of it is anxiety; more to come as she learns more, but tonight when I started whining, she brushed me for a long time. It was soothing and she scratched places I can't reach. I think it made me feel better. Dogs who are down in the hind legs can't scratch their neck or chest so it feels really good to have it done for you.

Now if Tipper would just leave us alone and not try to get brushed at the same time, I'd like it even better. Dad and Mom are proud of the Wake Forest High School Football team who won the state championship today. I've learned some things about football by listening to Dad as he watches. I've learned that "No, no no no" means his team didn't do something right, and "Yes, yeah!" means something good. So, Mom says that Santa is coming next weekend. I thought he was already here ... I think she's forgotten that he is standing beside the fireplace and he has his hand on his hip like he's surprised she forgot. Please remember to bring your fur babies in out of the cold. If you are cold, so are they.

December 18, 2016

I am in the same spot as I was last night! Slight difference in temperatures today and it was almost balmy. So..... no fire in the fireplace tonight. Dr. Ruth comes this week for my acupuncture and I am looking forward to it. I always feel so much better after she comes. Mom also suggested I let you know about Amazon Smile. If you order from Amazon, make sure to go to the Amazon Smile website where you can order and some of the money goes to a non-profit of your choice. It's an easy way to make sure your purchasing has power to help. We want to send blessings and thanks to all of you during this Christmas and New Year season.

I hear the word "Peace" a lot in the music being played in our house. Mom says many of the songs have been around for hundreds of years and they were wishing for peace even then. Peace must be a wonderful thing but extremely hard to get since the songs and wishes of the season are for peace. I wonder what it takes for so many people to want it and not have it. I have peace. I love my family and I am loved. I am not angry about my hard past, just really thankful it is over. I guess I sort of live in the moment and spend most of my days being grateful. I hope each one of you has peace in your life and that if you don't right now, you know that every day is a new beginning and peace for you will come. St. Francis of Assisi said it best.

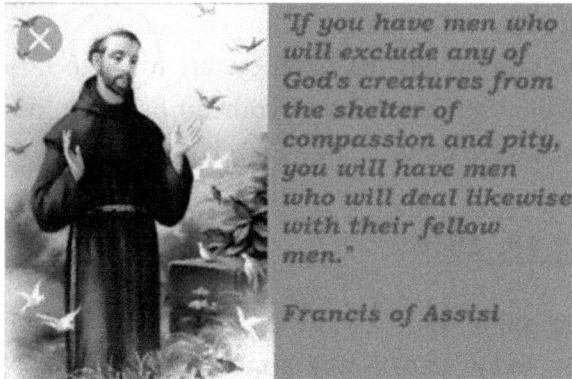

'If you have men who will exclude any of God's creatures from the shelter of compassion and pity, you will have men who will deal likewise with their fellow men.'

Francis of Assisi

December 19, 2016

There were a lot of new smells coming from the kitchen today. My human sister Rachael was helping Mom and they were using a buzzy thing and a lot of bowls and then putting things in that big hole in the wall where all the good smells were coming from. Mom says they were "baking".

Tomorrow, I've been told, is a trip to the big glass box where I get warm water sprayed on me and Mom rubs me all over. She calls it my Christmas bath. Looks like Annie and Buddy will be getting the same thing. One of the greatest things about Facebook friends is that you can take them with you wherever you go!

December 20, 2016

Ok so.... I don't know how the Life is Good advertisement made its way onto my page but I know I didn't put it there. Another new Facebook trick maybe?

So my bath has to be tomorrow because Mom says her plans went to hell in a hand basket. I don't know what that means, but I don't think it's good. Mom went to have her hair highlighted and came home with her hair a lot shorter. Dad likes it, but she always wears it up in a messy bun so it really doesn't look much different. Then they decided they needed to go to Costco so we had a boring afternoon. I got to be outside for quite a while when they came home.

December 21, 2016

I thought about not posting tonight but couldn't convince Mom so here we go. It seems one of the cats (I suspect Tipper) has her nose out of joint. She has intentionally peed on several things in the last two weeks. Let's see: Mom's tennis shoes in the closet, Buddy's bed, Sandy's bed and the rug inside the back door. All have been washed and treated but Mom has a nose for that in a nanosecond. I'm wondering what Mom is going to do about that bad behavior but I feel an exile to the upstairs room coming on for someone. Had no idea a cat could be so jealous or spiteful. No, Mom hasn't changed the cat litter to a different brand, and yes, the boxes get cleaned every day and we love Skout Urine Destroyer.

Mom is fit to be tied...whatever that means. Tipper has begun to snap at Lulu like an alligator if Lulu gets near her. Not good news for either one of them! Tipper, assuming it was her because she's the insecure one (Lulu is too daffy to be insecure), best mind her p's and q's and stop that marking behavior! Mom swore after the last two cats that lived to be 21 and 22 that she would not have cats again but that's another story for another night. Mom and Dad are so thankful for all the friends I have and for every good deed done because of reading one of my posts. Christmas blessings to all of you while much of the world prays for peace.

It is better to light just one little candle than to stumble in the dark. If everyone lit just one little candle, what a bright world this would be.

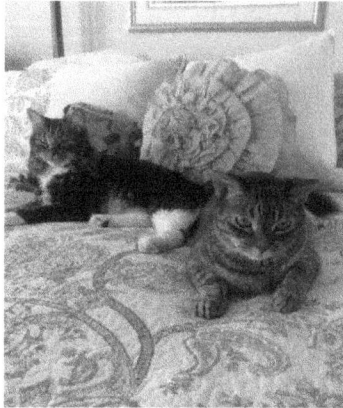

Lulu and Tipper

December 22, 2016

Life's unexpected gifts happened to me today and I was blessed with an early visit from Santa Claus! Then Dr. Ruth came and I had one of my best sessions ever and have been on the go or asleep the rest of the day. I had a great warm afternoon to tour the yard at my leisure and have had relaxed wonderful sleep. Tonight, I want to ask you something a little different. I'd like to ask you to send your strongest spirit and your healing, sustaining light to our wounded warriors and to our veteran service pups. Pray for their strength, their healing of body and spirit and join me in asking for blessings on them.

December 24, 2016

What a busy bee my mom was today. Meanwhile, I had a routine day and Tipper went to the vet. She got shots and pills for a possible infection and the lab work will be back Monday. Mom and Dad put Annie on a diet and are cutting back on her food intake. She is a butterball! The man beside the fireplace, named Santa Claus, is still watching so we are all on good behavior. The smell of food in that hole in the kitchen wall was mouth-watering and all of us got doggie bones tonight as an early Christmas present. I think I really like this time of year with all its sparkly things and wonderful smells.

We heard today about a senior age dog that was surrendered to a shelter because he had health problems and they didn't want to deal with him. The shelter put out a plea for a home and an angel came along and he was adopted. Other good news was that our friends **at Trio Animal Foundation** were able to pull 5 more dogs from high kill shelter because of the donations they received. There are hundreds in shelters this Christmas and our prayer is for more people to become enlightened by what it means to adopt or foster a needy dog or cat. Mom and Dad want you to know that not only have I changed their life, but you all have helped change mine. May each of you share the joy of Christmas day with love and peace in your heart.

December 25, 2016

Merry Christmas! All is warm and merry and bright except Mom and she's worn slam out! Sending love to all and hope your day tomorrow is full of knowing you are loved. Warm hugs to all!

We are celebrating on the 27th, so Sandy and Annie and Buddy and Lou Lou and Tipper will all get their Santa Claus and stockings that day. We normally travel back to Richmond, VA for the 24th and 25th to be with the rest of my family.

December 27, 2016

SANTA CAME TO SEE ME!!! We were wild and caused a bit of commotion but you should see my new toys! Annie started barking when she saw her stocking and all of us were so excited. I got toys and squeaky balls and a huge bone and I am so happy I don't know which to go after first or next! So here is a picture of us!

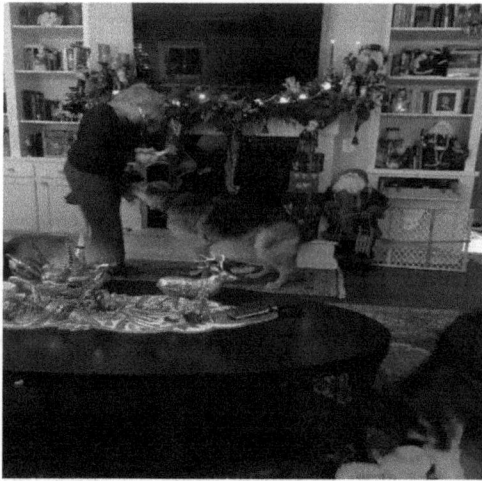

December 28, 2016

Not only did Mom and Dad spoil us on Christmas but today, I had a luxurious visit to the big glass box. Mom massaged me and got my tummy so pink and clean! I've been weary all day after the bath and Santa excitement! My wonderful Facebook family continues to amaze me and my mom and dad with all the love and support sent our way. Can you believe I actually had a real Christmas for the first time in my life. I had so many pups while I was being abused and neglected and I hope with all my heart they are safe and loved. Can't help but think about that every now and then.

We will celebrate my one year of being in my home in the third week of January. My rescue has been a blessing beyond measure, and Mom and Dad say I am a huge blessing to them. They say loving me has made their hearts grow. So, my work in making people aware of Saving Them All and don't shop, adopt... my work continues. With your love, the miracle goes on!

December 29, 2016

It was a restful day for me. Mom and Dad had errands to do, so I took advantage of the quiet and napped. This was AFTER I got Mom up at 5:00 a.m. but she's just glad I still let her know I need to go outside. Christmas lights are still shining brightly at our house so we can welcome in a year I never thought I'd see. It's just so amazing that I have this wonderful life with love and kindness from so many people. You know, North Carolina is not a no-kill state and still has so many counties with high-kill shelters. Plus, North Carolina discriminates against so many breeds and so many are put down because of their breed. So Mom has an idea but she needs your help. She is thinking about publishing all my Facebook posts since the very beginning of me telling my story.

In order to do this, she needs help figuring out how to print out each post or the contents of the whole page. Then, she could edit it with spelling corrections and so forth and promote it for raising funds to help the right people or right organization to change things in North Carolina. She would probably seek the help of Best Friends (see www.bestfriends.org) because they've been so successful in doing this all over the country. So we need your help in figuring out how to print out all of my posts. It's a lofty goal but it needs to start somewhere and I figure it might as well start with me. With all of you as my family and the best network ever, surely this could be done. Any and all help/suggestions are welcome because we don't know how to do it.

December 30, 2016

I've tried the links for compiling a book... difficulty is that my mom's personal page is her main Facebook page and my story is on another one of her pages... Mom copied and pasted many of the beginning posts but it is tedious, so she needs to look on Facebook on the computer and copy posts from there...will try it this weekend. Mom plans to contact Best Friends next week for some guidance. She will let all of you know if there are things she needs help with that can be done via Facebook or messaging. It's going to be a monumental task, so she needs a plan.

Mom and Dad celebrated their anniversary today. Friends came over and I was the star of the party! Tomorrow is game day so we will be fire side watching! As this year draws to a close, I want to thank each and every one of you for reading my posts, for sharing them, and for helping to awaken so many people to the abuse and neglect so many dogs and animals endure. Thank you for helping with every share you post because we have reached over 30,000 people during the last year. It's unbelievable, and as I lie here on my warm comfy waterproof bed, I pray each of you enjoys peace and love during the coming year. Our hearts are full, we are blessed.

January 1, 2017

A rainy cloudy January 1, 2016, but the fireplace is going and my tummy is full and we are all warm and safe. We heard today about a German Shepherd from Southeast German Shepherd Rescue that got adopted last night and then ran away last night...... she's all black and very skittish due to being abused and neglected so they are organizing a search for her. And believe it or not, it's in Wake Forest, where I live.

By the way, Tipper is fine and all her tests came back just fine so they treated her for a UTI and it seems to be a jealousy marking she's making. This does not make Mom or Dad happy.

However, we have been lucky enough to discover Skouts Honor pet odor and stain destroyer, and it works!! Better than anything we have ever tried!! It comes in several formulas so check it out!

Mom has started taking down the sparkly things....... she and Dad will be going up and down the stairs for the next few days putting it all away. I rather like it and wouldn't mind it being out all year.

Things Mom said today:

I wish I could wave a magic wand and all this stuff be packed and put away.

If I could invent Christmas lights that were guaranteed to burn for 10 years, I'd be a millionaire.

How can there be so much dog hair when I just vacuumed last night? (This is a dead giveaway about how exciting their New Year's Eve was).

So if you have momisms to share, please do and maybe we will compile them all.

2017 – The Living Part Two

"If you have a dog, you will most likely outlive it; to get a dog is to open yourself to profound joy, and, prospectively, to equally profound sadness."

~ Marjorie Gardner

January 1, 2017

Happy New Year!!

A short message tonight: Mom is thankful for pee pads and extra blankets and my diapers because I'm wetting my bed now. Say prayers this is a phase. Thank you!

January 2, 2017

This house is a WRECK! Decorations are spread out everywhere to be packed and Mom was so busy today she didn't run the vacuum even once!

We have a few days of the bleaks with dreary, chilly weather. We are all lazy and ready for some sunshine!

I played ball today! My version of playing ball: Mom or Dad throws the ball, I try to catch it without moving, Mom or Dad retrieves the ball, and we repeat. I do catch it sometimes and am most proud of myself when I do.

Update: Jewel has been found! There was a search for the lost black German Shepherd named Jewel today. She is afraid of people, won't come when called, and does like other dogs. She was lost off of Highway 98 here in Wake Forest near the Bowling Green subdivision.

I am so happy to hear that some of you have adopted a pet, that some of you have started to volunteer at shelters, and that you are helping spread the word about animal abuse.

I was dismayed to learn that Atlanta Falcons honored Michael Vick and Mom was furious. He was a thug when at Virginia Tech and then Mom got to work with some of his victims when she volunteered at Best Friends Animal Sanctuary in Utah. Mom vows never, ever, to watch the Atlanta team again, and she did the same thing when he was on the roster with the Eagles. If you could have seen the dogs he fought and abused it would break your heart. Such a poor choice by Atlanta to honor a felon convicted of animal cruelty! Please share this so people around the world will know what the Falcons did!

January 3, 2017

Proin! Seems to be helping a great deal! So far no wet beds today. I had a wonderful hour in the sunshine in the backyard with Annie and Buddy and I actually pooped and peed by myself holding myself up with all my might! I got lots of praise from Mom and it made me feel pretty good about myself. The fresh air made me perky! Good thing I got it today because cold frigid weather and snow is headed our way on Friday.

Mom and Dad took down all the outdoor sparkly lights today, and the man beside the fireplace has gone up the chimney I guess.

So after another few days of putting away all the decorations, Mom will be looking into how to publish my story to benefit homeless shelter dogs.

And please don't forget to watch Guardians of the Rescue on Animal Planet this coming Saturday night at 10:00 p.m.! A classmate of Mom's and Dad's from college, who was also an accomplished FBI agent, is part of this new show about stopping animal abuse! His name is Joaquin Garcia, and he also wrote a book called MAKING JACK FALCONE.

January 5, 2017

Another successful no wet bed day! Mom and Dad had to run to Richmond, VA, and back so my favorite Vet Tech, Lexi came and let us go out. Dad had a tooth implant issue (I don't even pretend to know what that means) but it turns out he really does not. When in doubt always seek another opinion!!!!! So all the hubbub about the expected snow has successfully made all the humans run for loaves of bread and milk like we will be house bound for days. Turns out it's going to be much ado about nothing since we will have sleet and not snow. Mom said this would happen. (She had to get her two cents in). Anyway, we are all gathered around the fireplace and enjoying a lazy evening. And just FYI, I held myself up again today to poop! I know it seems ridiculous that that is such a big deal but when I've required help with a harness every day for almost a year, this is quite an achievement. We are celebrating all of my achievements and spending time marveling at the generous wishes and support from all my Facebook family. I am so thankful for every post and every comment and for every morning I wake up in my home.

‚January 8, 2017

And…drum roll please! We have RAIN. We have sopping wet trees and bushes and yard. I do hate wet feet and am grateful for my nice new boots so I don't get wet feet or get that stuff on the sidewalk in my paws! Mom grew up at the foot of the Blue Ridge mountains where a foot of snow was no reason to even call off school. People never scrambled for bread and milk because they stayed prepared. So Mom and Dad went for regular grocery shopping today and not only was there a run on bread and milk but cucumbers too!

Tonight I am hoping you will send all your prayers and healing to the victims and their families and all those who were terrified in the Florida shooting. Even with all the prayers for Peace during Christmas, and the millions of prayers in Christmases of hundreds of years, it seems we will never understand the darkness that can overcome a soul. So I am thankful that we can find rays of light through sharing love.

January 9, 2017

Yes we are iced/snowed in. Sorry no posts but Mom has the full-fledged flu. I'll be back after I finish watching over her.

January 11, 2017

We are back and Mom wants to thank all of you for the good wishes. Dad has been on double duty since Friday night. Mom's "flu" was aching, fever, chills, no intestinal stuff and no sore throat or cold. Very odd! So she looked up the side effects of the meds she was put on for the tooth saga...300 mg Clindamicin. Sure enough, fever, chills, aches, all side effects, so she stopped taking it and by 1:00 today was out of bed and doing laundry and packing up Christmas stuff. That stuff is wicked!

We have 3" of ice topped with 2" of snow so sweet Dad has treated the back walkway and made a path for us to the yard. It's still very, very cold so no melting yet and I'm a bit slippery but doing ok. Dad started letting me go on my own out into the yard and I have done ok. All I must have is help with the steps. My new boots are going to be in use for a while since it will be cold, wet and slushy for a while outside.

We are predicted to have temperatures of 69 to 70 by Friday, so this is crazy weather.

We have heard of lost dogs and kitties in this weather and pray they find a warm spot and safe place until help comes. Please don't pass by a stray if you see one. If the dog or kitty won't come to you call the nearest veterinarian to find out the name of the local rescue who has resources to trap and save these babies.

January 12, 2017

It's my first re-birthday! Here's to a year in review and Dr. Ruth was here today to make this day special!!!

Mom and Dad and Dr. Ruth spent some time this morning marveling at what I have overcome and being thankful for this miracle. Dr. Ruth West admitted that when she first saw me she thought I was a short timer.

We all want to take this special day to thank each of you for reading about me, for talking about me, and for praying for me through your energies and empowering prayers. Who knew at the beginning of this journey my posts would be read at some point or another and I've been able to touch the hearts and minds of so many? I am a miracle. Every day and hour I have lived these past 365 days is a miracle. There is no doubt that you all made this happen. You lift me up, you give us strength and you are our personal heroes for believing in me. The God in each of you has found its way to my heart and soul and to the heart and souls of my entire family. We all feel incredibly blessed. Mom and Dad want to thank you for being their cheerleaders and my followers through so many ups and downs and through the days to come. Every dog, every creature deserves the best humans have to offer. Sometimes the best is a simple pat on the head or a prayer.

Most of all, we want to thank you for sharing my story of neglect, abuse, and rescue. Every time you share it, the chances are increased that someone will wonder about that poor dog chained in the rain or that skinny kitty climbing out of a dumpster.

January 13, 2017

And so I begin my second year of living in a warm comfy home with my own "your bed" and loving family.

For anyone new or relatively new to my page here is a recap of how I got here. In December of 2015, I was confiscated by law enforcement from being kept in unsanitary outdoor conditions, most likely chained. I weighed 57 pounds and had no fur from my shoulders to the tip of my tail and none under my chin to my tummy. I was covered in mange and my toenails were so long I could not stand up. I was estimated to be 10 years old and on the list to be put to sleep. A kind volunteer at the shelter saw something in me that wanted to live and contacted Southeast German Shepherd Rescue to see if they could possibly save me. That kind lady's name was Sandra and when SEGSR (Southeast German Shepherd Rescue) was finally able to pull off a last minute foster family, I was taken by them to a veterinarian and released to my now forever parents. It looked doubtful that I would survive but they were determined to let me have a clean bed and be as comfortable as they could in my last days. The Rescue had named me "Sandy" after the lady at the shelter.

After months of 24/7 care and trips to specialists and testing and treatment, 2 baths weekly, and special supplements and diet, I began to thrive. I do have special needs since I have severe spondylosis and degenerative myelopathy and have little use of my back legs. But through determination and love I am happy and able to get around enough to support myself to drink and occasionally to use the bathroom. I have wonderful wheels for walks in good weather and I have the warmest blankets and coats you could imagine. I have special boots for walking so I don't scrape my feet because I drag them some. Most all of these wonderful things were sent to me as gifts from many of you who follow my journey.

I get a regimen of meds and supplements that Mom and Dad credit for me being mobile at all. I now weigh 78 pounds and my coat is beautiful. I have a sister, Annie, and a brother, Buddy and two kitties, Tipper and Lulu.

With the help and support of some of my friends I am able to have acupuncture every two weeks which keeps the nerve connections working in my hind end. This helps me with incontinence and walking!!!

I am the face of Rescue. I would be dead if not for people who worked to save me and find me a home. Caring for me would have been a huge burden on my folks financially but we were urged to create a GoFundMe account which has made all of the medicines and veterinary visits and diagnostic tests and therapy and wheels and supplements and even yoga mats possible. Yes, our house is lined with yoga mats so I don't slip on the hardwood floors.

I have just celebrated my first Christmas in a warm loving home.

They don't know how old I am, but I can tell you that I would not have lived through another freezing winter or sweltering summer. I was so broken and my spirit was almost ready to give up. Then love came along and here I am.

Our mission has just begun and it seems Mom's passion for animals and her love for writing will result in an effort to help the abused, the neglected, the forgotten, the lonely, and the scared sick pups and kitties that populate our country.

We will keep my candle lit to light others as we venture into the second year of my re-birth, my rescue and my forever family.

We love you.

Sandy

January 14, 2017

It was a spring day in January today! Mom and Dad put me in my wheels and off we went on the longest walk I've had in months. So tonight I am very tired but happy. Thank you to all my FB family for the good wishes and blessings for my second year of really living.

Mom and Dad and I have a big task ahead of us to gather all my posts…we hope to get started next week. In the meantime, take a moment and invite your friends to see my page, and if you are following other rescue efforts like we do, share the pages!!

Best Friends and Bob's Shoes have a goal and all of us can help! BY 2025 ALL TREATABLE AND HEALTHY SHELTER ANIMALS WILL BE ADOPTED AND NOT KILLED!

January 15, 2017

Two notable things for today:

I went and got the ball and took it to Mom and dropped it in front of her!

My anxiety at night did not happen last night because I had been for a walk, so I'll be exercising more often.

Mom has a sinus headache tonight so we will post more tomorrow!

January 16, 2017

I made sure to wake Mom up at 6:30. Didn't want to shirk my normal duty! But she went back to bed and Dad got up to feed us. Then he went back to bed. That didn't suit me so I whined until Mom got up and kept us company.

Mom read that dogs with DM and spinal issues get anxiety at night so night before last when I went for a walk in my wheels, I didn't whine and act anxious. So, after dinner tonight Mom and Dad took all of us for a walk. I WALKED TWO BLOCKS! I am not whining…too tired! Mom and Dad were happy with how I wanted to go once in my wheels!

We are thankful for the fair weather and no ice!

Dad was busy carrying boxes to the attic today and all the sparkly Christmas things are packed away. I will go for my check-up sometime the next two weeks. In the meantime, Mom and Dad are going to start copying all my posts to begin the work ahead.

Reminder: Mom wants me to remind you to take all your old sheets and blankets and bath mats to your nearest veterinarian or shelter. They always need them.

January 17, 2017

I had visitors tonight for dinner! Bella and Bucket came with sis for dinner with Mom and Dad. Big sis works in the field of genetics and the conversation was way over my head …… chromosome thingies and noninvasive prenatal testing and spectrum disorders and all kinds of weird things I've never heard of.

I tried to herd Bella around the room but she can be more agile than me, but it surely was good exercise.

We are thankful today. Thankful for our many blessings and reminded of the powerful energy that is above and around us if we choose it. It is a big week for us in the United States, for we will inaugurate a new president. Our family prays for his guidance and wisdom. We pray for all the citizens of the United States that they too will be guided and show wisdom. We pray for all nations and all people to know the power of love and healing.

January 19, 2017

Mom got up this morning and stumbled around looking for her slippers because we awoke rather early. It was so early that I didn't even want my breakfast and we all went back to bed. By 8:00 I was hungry and so we got up all over again. My latest display of attitude is about the Ginger Harness. If Mom or Dad says it is potty time and I really don't want to go out, if Mom or Dad picks up the Harness, I go the opposite direction and drop myself into being dead weight on the floor. I think Mom figured it out tonight. My stubborn streak is showing. Mom and Dad think my stubborn streak is possibly the only thing that kept me alive before I was rescued, so they try to be very patient with me. Today was laundry day for all of our blankets so tonight we are on fresh beds and down for the count. We have another idea about how we can help lost pets. If you know of a shelter or a veterinary practice that offers free or discounted chipping please post it on my page. Mom will compile a list and post it to be shared with my many friends who we hope will post it again and again.

January 20, 2017

Another walk on my wheels and I did the whole block! It really does help with my night time anxiety. I use all four of my legs when in my wheels so I wear boots on my hind feet to keep from scraping them. I only wish I could walk that far without wheels, but then again, I'm lucky to be walking at all.

By the way, my sleeping buddy in yesterday's picture is Annie. She and Buddy always come along on my walks.

Mom wants me to make sure you know about SOI dog Foundation in Thailand that works to keep dogs off of the meat market. You can find out more on their Facebook page.

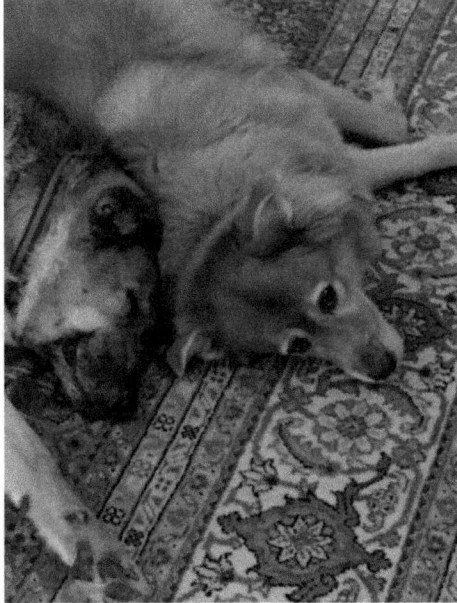

January 22, 2017

So here are a few things I've heard Mom and Dad say about the history that happens tomorrow:

- I want this pilot to fly this plane!
- The office of The President of the United States deserves respect.
- We each have a choice about the words we use, the hope we spread and the negative or positive energies that take up our brain space.
- I love this country and am grateful to be an American.

- It doesn't matter if you are red, yellow, black or white in the end...... it matters how you live your life.
- Prayer, Hope, and Goodness topped with wisdom has saved Sandy...we don't need to be afraid, we need to be proud of our country.

So, wave a flag tomorrow and be thankful for every opportunity to touch someone's or some dog's life in a positive way.

January 22, 2017

Things I am thankful for:

My sight

My "your bed"

My medicine

My food

My mom

My dad

My siblings

My kitties

My booties

My wheels

The yoga mats Mom uses on the floor

Water

My legs

My fur

Saving Sandy   Diana B. Mahoney

My clean skin

My acupuncture

My massages

My veterinarian

My pet sitter

My yard

Sunshine

The fire in the fireplace

Kind words

Soft pats on the head

Treats

Rugs to lie on

My Facebook family

My GMM

Mom always says when you are feeling bad, count your blessings.
I was tired today but ready for a good day tomorrow

January 23, 2017

A rainy sleepy day but Mom washed all the beds and blankets and
even cleaned all the carpet!

Tomorrow, I get a bath in the big glass box!

Thanks to all for the blessings and prayers always! We will have a longer post tomorrow... and we've begun the printing and editing of my posts!

January 24, 2017

We have had a couple of very gloomy wet days and Mom thinks maybe that's why I'm not up to par. I have had more trouble getting around the past few days and my front feet have begun to sort of paddle when I walk. I can't walk in a straight line because my back end is so weak on the right side and I tend to move more towards the left. We have Dr. Ruth coming on Tuesday so Mom and Dad will see what she thinks. I've been very fussy in the evenings and we haven't been able to walk because of the weather. Mom will talk to Dr. Ruth about my anxiety too. I did play ball with Mom early this afternoon...I lie there and she throws it so I can catch it. She gets more exercise than I do because although I am pretty good at catching, I can't move much while lying down so she's the retriever. Mom and Dad are huge believers in the quality of life and they watch mine very closely. Tonight in our area, two beautiful huskies are missing and feared stolen. We are praying for their safe return. If you see something, say something. It applies to animals too!

January 25, 2017

Yes, Dr. Ruth came today and I had a wonderful acupuncture session. I promptly took a nice long nap afterwards and was totally relaxed. Dr Ruth says my front paws may be beginning to lose muscle tone and to keep me walking as much as possible. She says I am still full of spark and life and we are doing all the right things. She did recommend more shoulder massages so Mom will be doing those. We talked about Adequan but it is more for synovial fluid assistance than for degenerative disc disease. Staying active is a key to my feeling less anxiety and sleeping better. My session was soothing and I yawned and yawned because it relaxed me so much.

We will be having our big bath day tomorrow because Mom ran out of time this week. I also am quite ready for a nice warm bath and lying in front of the fire to dry off. Mom says her eyes are crossing and we have to go to bed. Love to all and thank you for your continued prayers.

It's very late but wanted my FB family to know I did ok today. Still slow and hard to get around but I did ok. Glad Dr Ruth is coming in the morning at 10.

"When all the world is fast asleep

And shadows from my past creep into my dreams, I run.

My four legs carry me through soft green grass, through crunchy fall leaves and deep winter snow.

My nose twitches as I smell the rain and the spring blossoms.

I run. Free of pain, I sniff and shake my head when bees buzz.

In my dreams."

Sandy

January 27, 2017

I am grateful for today. Today I was able to walk around the yard in beautiful weather. I did my dog thing and enjoyed every sniff and every wobbly step. I am thankful for a wonderful home and good meds and my your beds and my Annie and Buddy and Tipper and Lulu. I love my mom and dad and there's no better place than lying on their feet. We will concentrate on our blessings and keep our determination.

Mom and Dad are amused at my stubborn ways and know it is my stubbornness that has helped me survive. Life was just fine for today.

Praying tonight for all the dogs with illness and spinal issues, all the hungry and cold pups, all the captive pups in puppy mills. Please say a prayer for them and send them your healing light

January 28, 2017

Oops. I missed a night last night. We had such gorgeous weather yesterday and I spent a lot of time outside. Even got to lie on the sidewalk in the sun. Tomorrow, Mom and Dad will put the Help Em Up harness on me for two or three days to give my shoulders a rest. I pull my body weight with my front end and can't put much weight at all on my back legs. Dr. Ruth says that North Carolina State Veterinary School is doing a study on "down dogs" ... that means they are studying spinal diseases that are causing dogs to lose the use of their back ends and front legs.

I'm going to get Mom to see if there is a way to follow what they are doing on line. I'm posting a video that will make you laugh. Mom and Dad were watching an historical piece on tv about the Holocaust so you might want to turn the volume down while watching the video. This my kitty, Lulu with a piece of plastic attached by static to her tail.

January 29, 2017

It was really a January day here! Cold in the morning and windy. Mom had to go to a dress rehearsal this morning and she looked like Nanook of the North all bundled up. Ok, I don't really know who Nanook is, but it sounds good...I think I may have heard it from someone

Dad says there is a lot of unhappy people around the world and I just wish I could tell some of them how happy they should be for

shelter and being able to walk ...... but that's maybe why I'm here......
to encourage, to spread hope, to show unconditional love. Maybe I am
a messenger or at least an example of how love overcomes the
shortcomings of humans.

January 30, 2017

Dad and all of us except Mom got up at 5:30 this morning so effective
asap I will be taking myself to bed. Of course, you already know that
if I get up, I demand that someone stay awake with me, so Dad didn't
go back to bed. Never mind that in an hour, once he's fully awake, I
will lie down and take a nice morning nap. Thank you all for your kind
comments and the love you share with me and my family. Who knew
that an old crippled German Shepherd could find so much love and
support and reach the thousands of people?

Do you realize that if every single person who looked at my posts
even once... if every single person helps directly or indirectly to save
a suffering fur baby, we'd save over 15,000 of them! That is
staggering. I am so grateful! Oops...that would be 27,000 saves. Mom
just checked the statistics. Think of it!

January 31, 2017

Mom got up early with me today. It was pretty cold at 5:30. I ate and
let her go back to bed.

I have a very special request tonight. Please go to Trio Animal
Foundation's Facebook page to see this pitiful baby they rescued
tonight. Please pray hard for her and send her all the love and healing
she needs. Her name is Liz and she needs all of us!

My sincere gratitude and much love,

Sandy

February 1, 2017

Note to self: it's ok to wake mom up as long as Dad gets up when she goes back to bed.

I felt happy today. It was warmer and the air was fresh and breezy.

Mom trimmed Buddy's feet and his coat. Annie was on the list for being next but escaped for today.

Tipper is in trouble again for not using her box...it had been determined by the vet that she has no UTI and just has an attitude problem which doesn't make Mom happy. All of us get along with each other so well and we share Mom and Dad, but Tipper thinks she owns Mom. We are all glad Mom found Skout's Honor to put on the carpet! It really works.

We have lots of things to be thankful for and I am so glad to have the chance to be thankful!

February 2, 2017

Well, as some of you may have noticed, many of my posts are written in the late evening/early morning.

We were all informed today that Mom will be on a mission to live a healthier way by going to bed at a decent hour. The goal is to be in bed no later than 11:30, with 11:00 p.m. being the best. So there may be some nights when my posts are delayed until the next morning.

I don't know who she thinks she is fooling. She's been a night owl since she was in her 30s (so at least a few years now, bahahaha). Her mom was and her sister is, so we will just see how this goes.

Keep in mind she did not consult with me about this decision. Therefore I won't take any responsibility for her success or failure at this new goal.

Looks like spring here.... daffodils are really confused and blooming already and so are the redbud trees. Even saw forsythia today. Punxsutawney Phil better watch out! I may take his job!

February 4, 2017

I had to get my rabies vaccination today and I weighed in at 80 pounds. Wow. Mom says I have to lose 3 to 4 so I stay on my feet. My vet, Dr. Thames, is amazed at how different I am and is such a good partner with my parents in my treatments. We are so blessed to have such a wonderful veterinarian just one mile from our house!

Mom looked back through all my records today and it has been such a miracle that I am here, that I enjoy life and that I have so many people who love me.

I am a wobbly girl but my stubbornness has served me well for surviving and even thriving.

So when you think you've come to the end of your rope, tie a knot and hang on!!

February 5, 2017

Mom and Dad had the thrill of seeing and hearing the St Olaf Choir and orchestra! It was a wonderful thing for Mom to be able to do because she listened to their Christmas program every Christmas Eve for years so it was really special to her.

I've had a bout again with diarrhea so I'm back on some things to calm my tummy down. Mom thinks it's because of the stress of going to the vet but I ate well and wanted to play ball. I just have a plain old sensitive tummy.......

And, what the heck is a Super Bowl? Dad wants to know what the menu is....... I think he wants Mom to fix the traditional buffalo chicken dip. It is a football tradition they have and after what I've been told is the last game for an eternity, no buffalo dip until the eternity is over (August).

The message from the St. Olaf choir was to be compassionate, to do everything we can to honor life and to love one another. That's a tall order for all of us, and Mom especially because she is so against animal cruelty and puppy mills and the horrible things people on this earth do to animals. So, I guess she's got to practice more.

February 7, 2017

Mom is an hour behind...behind going to bed. I am feeling better today and am on food for sensitive stomachs. And..... we've added Proin to my meds to keep me from leaking at night.

I'm looking forward to the nice weather this week and hoping I can get back in my wheels for a bit. I got my nails trimmed when I was at the vet and need to get a couple of pounds off so I can walk better. Can you believe it?

Tonight I am thankful for my clean "your bed" and for things being back to normal.

Still praying for Liz at Trio Animal Foundation!

February 8, 2017

Yesterday got by us and we didn't do a good job posting. But the good news is that my digestive system is back to normal and I played ball with Mom for about 30 minutes last night. Keep in mind that my version of playing ball is I catch the ball while I am lying down and only when carefully aimed. But it did make me really happy!

We got some good news about Liz. She was able to stand by herself and is able to take in a couple more tablespoons of food!

Today was ear cleaning day and if I could run away from Mom when she comes with the cotton pads, I would. But my ears are in good shape so just routine maintenance.

Mom and Dad are off today to see the orthopedic surgeon at Duke for Dad's final visit (we hope). How lucky and blessed we are to have had the Duke team surgeon as Dad's doctor!!!! Dad gets his card today that he'll have to carry because he sets off alarms at airports and secured retail stores due to the metal plate in his shoulder.

Keep prayers going for Liz! They really do work!

Loving the outdoors today! Daffodils are blooming and forsythia is budding!

February 7, 2017

I was the early riser today!!!! Mom got up with me at 6:00 and the sky was still dark and stars shining! I did let her go back to sleep for awhile but then of course I protested. So Dad got up to be with me. The big loud thing Mom pushes around the floor came out today so all of us had to move from room to room to stay out of the way. All of the plants and birds are very confused by our unusually warm weather.

Glad I'm not in the north east where it will be a snow blizzard this weekend! We will probably get rain. My Facebook family has become an integral part of our lives and we are so grateful for the connections we have made with all of you.

I continue to be able to wobble around but the odds of me being able to regain the full use of my back legs are very slim. My spine is affected by spondylosis which is like stenosis in people and it has caused permanent damage to my nerve endings. Everyone is amazed that I can still hold myself up enough to wobble from the bedroom to the den and kitchen but realistically, we know it is a matter of keeping the damage limited as long as we can and as long as I am happy and enjoying this wonderful life. So prayers for me to continue to be able to stand and control my body functions are what I ask for. I'm happy and I am enjoying life one day at a time!

Whoa! We are a cool 25 degrees now... it was 75 yesterday. It was spa day at our house and all of us got baths.... well, all of us except the kitties. I had a very long massage in nice warm water and fell asleep tonight right after dinner. I've just finished my last trip outside with my nice warm coat and am off to see the sandman. Dr. Ruth comes in the morning.

To my friends in the cold weather, please remember that no cat or dog can withstand the horrible cold without shelter. Bring them inside!

February 8, 2017

Woah! We are a cool 25 degrees now....... Was 75 yesterday. It was spa day at our house and all of us got baths...all of us except the kitties. I had a very long massage in nice warm water and fell asleep tonight after dinner. I just finished my last trip outside with my nice warm coat and am off to see the sandman. Dr. Ruth comes in the morning. To my friends in the cold weather please remember that no dog or cat can withstand the horrible cold without shelter. Bring them inside!

February 9, 2017

I wrote a very long post and forgot to post it so here's the short story:

Bella and Bucket came to stay for the weekend. It seems Bella thinks MY mom is hers and it made me really anxious but we are now exhausted from being in the yard most of the afternoon in 73 degree weather and worn out now. Mom tried to explain to me that Bella has been raised around her since she was 5 weeks old but that does not matter to me.

So if you need a Valentine, please think about getting one of the fur babies from your local shelter. There are some that have never known a home or had a Valentine and they would love you forever.

Here is a pic of Bucket and Bella:

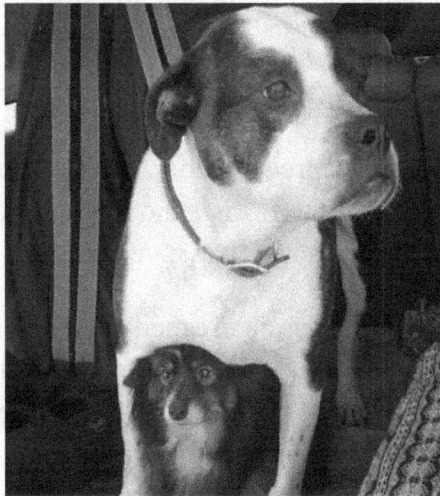

February 11, 2017

We spent an unusual February day in 80 degree weather! A cool breeze and a nice day in the yard! Bella is still getting the message some of the time. Mom seems to love on each of us so I'll get used to it. Last February was much colder and more rainy so we are happy with this warmth. It might mean an early spring and a very hot summer. We do need a nice hard freeze to keep the insects at bay. Mom and Dad are going to put me in my Help Em Up Harness for a few days to give my shoulders a rest from bearing so much of my weight. When I get tired, I have a hard time even getting up, but Mom and Dad help me know to wait for them to help me.

I've taught my family a lot about German Shepherd Dogs. We are constantly on alert when it comes to our home. We have anxiety when we feel like we can't do our job. Our eyes never miss a movement in the room. We are gentle giants until you mess with our people.

Tonight there are hundreds of people and dogs and cats and wildlife in danger of the dam breaking in California. Say a special prayer for their safety and for people to rally to help them.

February 14, 2017

So much for our 80-degree weather. Back into the 50s for us here. Mom worked today at the florist, and Dad was on duty all day. Bella and Bucket went home so we had a very relaxing afternoon.

We are so glad California escaped such a horrible catastrophe but we are not forgetting that so many are still in danger. Tonight, I am grateful for going to my "your bed," unafraid of anything. I am not afraid of being hungry. I am not afraid of being cold. I am not afraid of being beaten. I am not afraid of being unloved.

Happy Valentine's Day to all of you, my wonderful and faithful family. Make sure to tell your family that you love them and make sure to send your healing love to all the homeless and abused and starving fur babies.

My observations about Valentine's Day:

My mom and dad tell each other every day that they love each other.

My mom and dad tell all of us that they love use multiple times a day.

Mom says guys spend hundreds of dollars on flowers for their wives and girlfriends on Valentine's Day.

If they practiced saying "I love yous" every day then they could save a lot of money.

Valentine's Day is for anyone you love, not just wives or girlfriends or husbands or boyfriends.

AND... one more thing.

Why do people wait until Valentine's Day to actually buy flowers? They could order weeks ahead for delivery on the 14th.

Our Valentine's treat was having Ritz crackers instead of our regular treats. We were quite happy about it.

Anyway, tell your loved ones and friends you love them every chance you get. No one is promised tomorrow.

February 15, 2017

Oh, yes! Rumor has it! My only hope is that some way, this champion could become a champion to fight DM! Degenerative Myelopathy just has to be genetic and this dog could have a mission to be a Champion of the fight. Any Ideas?

Posting a tribute tonight that my mom saw on the Degenerative Myelopathy Facebook page. So beautiful I had to pass it on.

"2X Regional Champion "Debi" – First puppy born 1/5/2006 at 9:40 pm –last one left in her litter on this day at 2/1/17, 10:41 am…Left this earth at our favorite beach spot, overlooking Long Island Sound, on the sunniest, brightest day this winter, at low tide, surrounded by her baby sister Isabella, her loving care provider Anthony, her human mom and 2 dedicated friends, and her neurologist and his assistant who provided her with this selfless gift of Peace.

Debi was predeceased by her litter sister Dena on 7/18/2016 in the same location.

This beautiful, loving creature left with dignity. She was a fighter of Degenerative Myelopathy. She never gave up and protected me her whole life. She carried a stick, jute roll or towy, always. She was clear and never afraid. She was not sick a day in her life until this genetic disorder. I am numb, I am never going to have the working bond I had with Debi and Dena. I am forever in debt to my truly courageous son Anthony for all the care provided to these dogs in my absence and while there. How many 23-year-old kids would go to college, work 2 jobs, play gigs, and take care of not one but three dogs, 2 handicapped and indoor cats too!! Anthony, you are the strongest man I know, mentally and so brave. Watching what your mom has been through, your grandmother fighting cancer, AND taking care of the dogs at the same time while achieving good grades in college is just inconceivable. I wish there was an award I could pass to you for this!

To my Debi, I love you forever. I really don't know how I'm going to get thru these next days. Please enjoy our tribute to an awesome German Shepherd. I love you all for always being there for me and my dogs throughout their journey with Degenerative Myelopathy. I could not have gotten through this without all of you.

February 17, 2017

Mom is a night owl and not sticking to her plan. Anyway, we had a beautiful day and I had an upset stomach again. No reason since there's been absolutely no change in diet but I got chicken and rice anyway. I'm better tonight.

I've had a tough week getting around. My hind legs have been very weak and I can't support myself enough to go to the bathroom. We don't know if this is the progression or if I'll be strong in them again; we have to wait and see. My anxiety at night has increased and nothing soothes me. Mom came and laid beside me on the floor tonight and massaged my shoulders but I'm still anxious. I think it may have crossed Mom's mind that I'm beginning not to be having a good time in the evenings and how I have to lie around all day on my right side.

Tomorrow, we will try my wheels if my tummy is not a problem. I looked at Mom tonight with big question marks in my eyes when I was feeling so anxious and it just broke her heart. Tipper, the cat, came and curled up with me to offer some comfort and to get in on being brushed. She's not fooling anyone. It will be the Help Em Up Harness for a couple of days to give my shoulders a break. Mom wants to sit down and write a summary letter of my story to the owners of Rumor Has It so they understand the impact DM is having on so many innocent dogs. If she doesn't post a night or two, it's because she is working on the letter. Any and all advice for what she should say is welcome! I will post the website on how to contact them in tomorrow's post. That way if any of you feel so inclined as to ask them to read my story and help us stop this, I know it could be so helpful.

Thank you my FB Family.

February 19, 2017

I went out in the beautiful weather. My tummy is much better and Mom will talk to Dr. Ruth this week about my anxiety. Thanks for all the prayers and cheerful wishes! We are plodding ahead one day at a time. Remember to say a prayer for the pups and kitties who are so hungry tonight.

February 20, 2017

So I went to the vet today. Had a very rough night with being up every couple of hours needing to make a quick dash (ha ha) to the back door. We made it successfully once and I tried really hard to make it the other times. Anyway, I have an unbalanced bacteria count in my intestines so I am back on antibiotics and so far this evening I am better. Mom and Dad talked to the doctor about my whining and anxiety at night so we are trying a new medicine. Mom's not happy with it since it seems to knock me out, but will reduce it tomorrow. I did eat my dinner after being picky at breakfast. I am also up to 82.3 pounds so it's really diet time. I will be able to walk better if I lose 5 to 6 pounds.

Mom hasn't started on the contact for Rumor yet, but it is on her list. Thank you for always keeping me close in your hearts and for all the prayers! We are thankful for veterinarians!

February 20, 2017

OK, I'm pretty laid back today. The meds have stopped my intestinal stuff but have also stopped everything else. We have gone outside numerous times today and we are thankful for the nice weather. Dr. Ruth comes tomorrow to do my acupuncture so Mom and Dad are going to talk with her about some of my meds. The list right now is so long!

- Gabapentin
- Tramadol
- Rimadyl
- Antibiotic
- B12
- EFAC
- Dasaguin
- Proin

And we are trying a low dose of Prozac for my anxiety which is over the top......melatonin did not work nor did anything else...yet.

We wish we could be more focused on saving dogs and cats and horses and other creatures but Mom says my health comes first.

February 22, 2016

I had the best day yesterday after Dr. Ruth came! I got up to go to the door to greet her! After my treatment, there was marked improvement in my walking! I walked into the kitchen, I was able to walk around the den without falling! And, things moved, if you know what I mean. I felt so much better afterwards.

Mom and Dad had a talk with Dr. Ruth and we decided to take me off of the Tramadol and to treat my anxiety with a low dose of antidepressant. We are on day two of no Tramadol and my evenings are now relaxed and I am peaceful. We have had to cut down on my food because I have to shed some lbs! Dr. Ruth agrees that it will be easier to hold myself up with a few pounds gone. Can you believe it? A year ago I was trying to gain weight.

I got a special card from my godmother today. Mom and Dad find it a blessing to know that if anything is needed my Facebook family always comes through! Once again, your prayers and support with your healing love have gotten me on my feet. It is miraculous what power there is in this family.

February 24, 2017

I am still tuned in to my internal clock and staying efficient at waking Dad or Mom so I can begin the day. However, I did refuse my food this morning, so to bribe me, Mom gave me all canned chicken and peas. My attitude is great and most of the day I'm happy. I get fretful at night and we are trying different things to help me. My shoulders and my front legs get very weary just going out several times a day. Thanks to all of you for pulling for me all the time. We are so thankful for the mild winter so I can enjoy the sun and lie down in the grass. So we continue into my second year having a soft place to lie down, food in my tummy, and shelter in this storm of life. We are blessed beyond measure for each day and for having all of you on this day-to-day journey.

February 26, 2017

All is well. Mom has been very busy – just got home late tonight due to rehearsal. Rest well and a more detailed update on me tomorrow. My love to all of you.

February 28, 2017

Ok. The past few days, or more like the past week, we have been trying Prozac as prescribed for my anxiety. Mom and Dad have carefully monitored my behavior and have now taken me down to one only at night. I'm not taking the Tramadol and today, I was almost back to being able to support myself in the yard. The higher dosage made me all wonky, and although it sure helped with the anxiety, it appeared to make me enjoy life less.

Today I tried to play with Annie for the first time in over a week, and I ate both meals! Dogs metabolize drugs differently from humans, and Mom and Dad are very aware of that, so they watch me as much as I watch them. Right now, we are having a big thunderstorm, and I am lying at Mom's feet as are all the other four-legged children. We had a windy day and I got to lie in the sun while Buddy barked just to hear himself and Annie poked around in the pine needles. We follow several animal rescues and we want to thank all of you who share the mission that together, we can save them all. XOXO.

March 1, 2017

I love the posts I get from my Facebook Family. So many times the prayers of this family have brought me through rough days and weeks, and I am proof that love and prayers and belief in the power of healing energies are what have kept a light shining in my eyes.

For the new readers of my page, I just want to assure all of you that Mom and Dad don't put me on any meds till they have been thoroughly thought out and researched and discussed with my doctors. I am blessed to see three veterinarians who monitor me closely and know my condition. I was fully evaluated at North Carolina State School of Veterinary Medicine a year ago and we have been blessed, through the support of many who love me, to give the best in meds and supplements and diet.   For the people who have asked what my treatment is, here is a list.

- EFAC – 1 capsule 2x a day
- Rimadyl – 1 pill 2x a day
- Gabapentin – 400 mg 2x a day
- Proin – 1 pill 2x a day

I was on Tramadol, but we stopped that two weeks ago and we haven't noticed a difference.

- Turmeric – 1 a day
- Vitamin Methyl B12 – 1x a day
- Probiotics = 2x a day

Lately, I've had to be on an antibiotic for the trouble I had with my intestinal stuff. I am off of it as of today. My spinal disease is unpredictable and fortunately, I can still manage to stand at the water bowl which is raised. I can't do any steps, and we use a Ginger Harness to help hold me up when I go outside. I was wetting my bed at night but now the Proin works really well.

I also have Eddie's wheels which we use on nice warm days and I can walk around for about 10 minutes. We use boots on my hind feet because I knuckle them under and drag them. We also have a Help Em Up Harness which I use every time I go to the vet and when my shoulders get tired.

I am so so blessed to have all the wonderful things I need because without the help of my Facebook Family, my mom and dad could not provide all of this. We are eternally grateful and the life I still enjoy is a gift from all of you.

A hint from Mom: Using a water proof cover on her bed is so helpful. We have two, so there is always one clean for the nighttime. Puppy pads are also helpful during the day if Sandy has some leaking.

March 2, 2017

Whoa!! Winter has reared its cold head again and Mom and Dad had to cover some blossoming plants tonight. I have had some pretty good days this week! I have some spark back and Mom and Dad think they've found the right combination of meds for the time being anyway. I am such a Shepherd!!!! If Mom goes into the bedroom, I follow to see what she's doing. If Dad goes into the kitchen, I watch every move he makes. And when Annie wants attention or when Mom talks to Buddy or Tipper or LuLu, I have to be right there in the mix. I am at this very moment watching the bedroom hallway to see if Dad is coming back out to the den. I am peering through the bottom of the coffee table.

March 4, 2017

My cousin Boz, my Auntie's GSD, has had a rough go of it. He had spinal surgery this past fall to repair a disc, then he tore his meniscus in his left hind leg when he fell so had to have surgery on that. He's been recovering nicely till today when he had two seizures. He has been on antibiotics because he developed a staph infection, and they put him on 300mg of Clindamycin twice a day. He had a seizure this morning early and another one early this afternoon and is in ICU at the Veterinary Emergency Center in Richmond, where his surgeons are. Please let us know if you've ever experienced this kind of thing from an antibiotic with your dog. My mom took it for a problem too, as some of you may remember. She had a terrible reaction to it (fever, chills, aches!!). Boz is 11 ½ years old and our family, as you might guess, is very attached to our pets. Please send prayers for Boz!!!!!

Later March 4, 2017

Thank you so so much for your prayers for Boz. He had a total of 3 seizures yesterday, two of which the bet stopped with intravenous Valium. He is now home and on some medicine called Keppra to prevent the seizures and will undergo neurological testing this week. He's pretty weak but he survived until they could get the seizures under control and now will see the specialists. It was very scary for him and his parents!

Meanwhile back at the ranch, Bella and Bucket are with me for a week while their mom is on business. We are all getting along just fine and are enjoying the fire tonight! Mom has come down with what appears to be a cold and she is not happy about it. Dad is working on the taxes and he is not happy about that either, and Mom is taking Zicam and Sudafed. A horrible thing happened in Richmond, VA…a poor puppy was abused and put into a suitcase into the river. You can to WWBT's website to watch the reward fund grow to catch the sub humans who did this. Pray that all these horrible people will be caught and punished.

March 6, 2017

I wrote a post, and somehow, it didn't. Mom has a bad sinus infection and the rest of us are fine. I'm only a little jealous of Bella, and as long as she doesn't lie on my bed, I'm ok.

We will post more tomorrow. Tell your fur babies that you love them!!

Annie says, "Yeah, I will lie here for just a few more minutes but then I'm moving!"

March 7, 2017

Our house is full of germs from Mom. She says her head feels as big as a watermelon but it sure doesn't look like one to me.

I did get to enjoy some time outside today because it has warmed up. We are working on keeping my leg muscles strong but the signal to make them work isn't getting from my brain down my spine so I'm a bit weaker. Bella keeps me moving around because she is a bed stealer. Mom has also had to yell at her for chasing the cats. If they wouldn't run, Bella wouldn't chase them but try telling that to a cat.

We have birds coming back now to build their nest in the little birdhouse out in back of the house. Our magnolia got ruined by the hard freeze but the snowball bush survived! Mom loves spring and to see the plants come back. Dad has already filed our taxes!!!! Yay!

Thinking tonight of the horrible people especially in states like Missouri and Alabama who run puppy mills and praying they can be stopped.

March 9, 2017

Mom is better and actually wasn't a slug today. Spring cleaning has begun so she was busy and kept Dad busy getting the office in order and the upstairs spotless. She says she has more to do.

We have very sad news today. My cousin Boz, a huge GSD, was diagnosed with a brain tumor that is large and in the frontal part of his brain. Boz was the inspiration for my mom and dad to become donors and fosters for German Shepherds. He is a gorgeous Black and Tan GSD who is loved dearly and has endured much this past year, coming through two surgeries with flying colors. My mom's sister has spent a solid year nursing him through surgeries and rehab with his back and his leg and he has been such a champ. Now this. My family is a strong believer in quality of life both for humans and dogs and all creatures.

It has been a lifetime journey of having pets that has taught us that keeping a suffering animal with us is selfishness on our part when they are not having a good time. I look back on my many pets and have some regrets that I didn't understand the importance of quality of life versus suffering. I am grateful that my journey has taught me this lesson, and my beloved pets will never be allowed to suffer due to my selfish wish to have them with me. Each pet has been a blessing to me, has taught me the true meaning of love and trust, and has helped me evolve to understand that our lives, our energies don't stop when our heart does. Please hold us close in your heart as my sister and her family make plans for their part at the end of this journey for Boz. He has taught great lessons.

Mom talked with her sister, Boz's mom, today and they are making sure the whole family gets to come and say their farewells to him. He had visits today and his beloved Pat came to see him. She always kept him whenever his mom and dad were out of town.

One of the things Mom talks about to most anyone who will listen, is the practice she found out about when she volunteered at Best Friends Animal Sanctuary in Kanab, Utah. Each dog has about 3 or 4 kennel mates. In their kennel, they each have a bed and openings to their yard outside. In the summer, they have their little swimming pools and most get walked each day by volunteers. The kennels are designed "in the round" so the dogs and caretakers have a lot of interaction.

Anyway, when a kennel mate crosses the bridge, usually they are at the veterinary facility on the grounds. The caretakers bring the dog back to the kennel after they are finished crossing, and place the dog on its bed. They believe it is so important for the kennel mates to understand that their friend has not just disappeared. They let the dogs smell and lick the friend who has passed. They then wrap the dog in its blanket. A burial ceremony in Angel's rest is held and all the staff and people who are there go to celebrate the gift of life and the existence of the animal who has passed. As the wind chimes in the trees make their music, each person, in a tradition much like Jewish burial, places a stone or small memento on the grave of the animal who has lived and gone on to the next energy.

The point in telling you this is that this is the way we do it in our family. Everyone gets a chance to celebrate and to grieve, all the 4 legged members and the 2 legged members. So that is how this will go, and Mom is so thankful to Best Friends for teaching her how important this is.

Thank you all our friends for the prayers and love you are sending our way. We know many, if not most of you have traveled this path before. The celebration is that we choose to commit ourselves to this when we love them.

Later

My wonderful supportive Facebook Family! We are grateful for the kindness you've expressed about my cousin Boz. He's going to enjoy the next few days, provided he does not have a seizure. He's being treated like a king and was so spunky today he even played with his ball. He has always loved the beach and he will get a final trip to see the ocean. His veterinarians at Sycamore Veterinary Hospital are on notice to attend to his every need.

Meanwhile, at our house, we all got our nails trimmed...... well, not ALL of us because you know how I am about the buzzy thing.
It is a time at our house for Mom and Dad to practice what they believe

and to be supportive in any way they know how. The energies of love and healing...

To each of you who has suffered the loss of a fur baby, may your hearts heal knowing:

All Things Bright and Beautiful, All Things Great and Small, All Things Wise and Wonderful, our Father Made Them All.

March 12, 2017

Today's update:

We had snow for two hours and it all melted 30 minutes after it stopped.

Boz had a good day actually playing ball and seeing some friends and family.

I had a good day. I have even learned to share my bed with Bella. Getting around is a little more difficult but it sure makes me determined when Bella is here.

Bucket has claimed a new spot on the big chair.

Mom's sinus infection finally broke loose!

And we have friends who want to find an Akita to adopt. They live in North Carolina so it needs to be a distance within reason and the adoptee must love other dogs and people.

Bella and Bucket go home tomorrow.

Tomorrow is pay it forward day, as declared by me, so open the door for someone, take a grocery cart from the parking lot to the store, call that person you've been meaning to call, thank the post person, pay the toll for the person behind you, pay the next person's fast food meal, take doughnuts to the office, speak to people on the elevator, say your prayers.

March 13, 2017

With the winter blizzard coming, please make sure you take your pets indoors. Check to make sure your neighbors are doing the same, and if you suspect an animal is being left in the cold, call animal control and report it. Two people near and dear to my mom have gone so far in blizzard weather to cut chains to free these neglected dogs or they would have frozen to death.

We have lots of cold rain and all of us are safe and warm inside. Bella and Bucket went home tonight so it's very quiet tonight.
Take an extra sheet or towel or blanket to your local shelter this weekend. They will need it.

March 14, 2017

Since Mom was under the weather last week, we've not been really working on getting more information from or to the GS who won the top award at the Dog show. Rumor has layers of people to go through it seems to make contact but we will begin again tomorrow. I am indeed slowing down and gradually becoming weaker in my hind legs. My shoulders get tired supporting the heavy weight of my chest and my hind end swings to the left as I walk. I want to keep you aware of my health but don't want to alarm you and don't want to give anyone false hopes that I will ever be able to walk well again. I am still a miracle dog because I am living a good life. I was rescued from the most horrible situation and in terrible shape, now I have a home, meals, beds, blankets, coats, wheels, and mess. Most of all, I have love and I give love. I am and always will be a miracle dog. Over 12 months ago, I was within 24 hours of death. Look at me now!

My cousin Boz is holding his own and has enjoyed the yard and his family the last few days. We trust that my auntie will make the decision about helping him over the Rainbow Bridge when it is time. All the vets who love him are on board and he has his very own vet tech who loves him like her own. He is in good hands.

So I am carrying on with my mission to increase awareness of DM, to help humans understand the responsibilities of rescue and to do my own little part of saving them all. Every now and then, my mom will weep for the cruelty that people impose on helpless dogs and animals. She feels so strongly that her journey has led her to understand the power of a relationship with a pet and that she must help make others aware and urge people to help. My parents are thankful every day for all the love sent our way and we want to always pass it on.

March 16, 2017

It's just downright cold here. I am restless from two days of being inside and not being able to lie out in the sunny side of the yard. It will make me double triple happy when spring really gets here to stay. Ok folks, I have a request. There is a very misguided man in Iowa who wants to make dog fighting legal. His name is Steve King and he is a United States representative, and I'd like you to go to his contact info and write to him about how much we are against his proposal! It needs our attention and support! Please take five minutes to tell him this is NOT OK!

Steve King has a Facebook page called Steve King. Here is what I messaged him:

Dear Mr. King,

You, sir, have poked the beast. Please clarify for me and the 16,000 Facebook followers my rescued dog has what you mean by legalizing dog fighting. I will refrain from further comment until I hear from you. If I do not, I will take your comments about legalizing dog fighting as your true position and will act accordingly. Thank you.

As you can see, Mom is on this like white on rice. You can go to www.dogtime.com and see how he explains his remarks. Meanwhile, I've had a good day, I ate well and even played ball for a few minutes. Your prayers are my healing!!!!!!!

March 17, 2017

Happy St. Patrick's Day! I can formally claim it because I am Sandy Mahoney! I had a better day today and enjoyed my special rice and chicken along with a little time outside. Mom says tomorrow is big glass box that rains on you day. She told me I smell like a dog. Ha! Hope all of you found time to message Steve King and give him your opinion of his stance on dog fighting. We have received not a single response from him.

Rescuing a pet is a big commitment, and we are so thankful for each one of you who has done it. We are also grateful for the volunteers among you and the ones if you who go the extra mile for those sad eyes and matted fur, for those starved and beaten. Blessings on you. Please read about the most recent Trio rescue, and many thanks for the St. Paddy's day gifts to my fund!!

March 19, 2017

I want you to know that when Mom took off my collar and told me it was bath time, I wobbled all by myself to the big glass box!!!! Mom always lines the bottom of the box with soft bath mats so I just went in and she didn't even have to put a leash on me to get me in!! I got a

35-minute complete body massage and loved the warm water! I've been so relaxed today after that.

Going online in a few minutes to get any updates on Mr. Steve King. Thanks to all of you who emailed and posted to his page and messaged him!!! More tomorrow!

Go to your search bar on Facebook and search for SteveKing@Steveking for congress. Please please message him. He wants to legalize dog fighting. I've told him Sandy has a large family, and he will hear from them.

My message:

Mr. King,

Since, by design or default, you have not responded to my message, I will be sharing your views on animal fighting with 16,000 followers on Facebook. You have chosen a path that I cannot abide by, and it is true that you can judge the character of a human being by the way he or she treats animals. To be a man of such opinions, you cannot possibly represent the humanity for which each of us is held responsible. You are not an honorable man or an evolved human being. You will reap what you sow.
https://www.facebook.com/pages/Steve-King/108036912558457

March 19, 2017

Steve King has a Facebook page under that name. Here is the message I sent him:

Dear Mr. King,

You, sir, have poked the beast. Please clarify for me and the 16,000 Facebook followers my rescued dog has what you mean by legalizing dog fighting. I will refrain from further comment until I hear from you. If I do not, I will take your comments about legalizing dog fighting as your true position and will act accordingly.

Thank you.

Diana

If he truly is for legalizing dog fighting, I will urge all of you to contact him. In the meantime, you can visit his Facebook page and decide how you'd like to approach this.

As you can see, my mom is fired up! And I had a much better day today. I ate well and played ball!!! Once again, your prayers are my healing!

Love,

Sandy

https://steveking.house.gov/

March 21, 2017

The revolving door at our house has spun in Bella and Bucket again. Their mom is reveling on business so here we go again. Don't know if any of you heard about the huge fire in Raleigh that burned a massive apartment building that was being built in downtown. My human sister's condo is right across the street of the block that it was in. Fortunately for her, the wind was blowing away from her building but the condos in the direction of the wind were burned and damaged all the way to the 15th floor. Windows melted, and a total of 10 buildings were involved. Every firefighter within a 30-mile radius of Raleigh was on notice because it was so massive. It took over three hours to control and three days of putting water on it. We are all feeling really blessed that she had no damage.

Mom thought her stupid sinus infections was gone then she got a cold that has now gone from throat and nose to chest. She is NOT a good sick person and gets very frustrated and bored about not being able to tackle the to-do list.

We were noticing today that when we moved into this house, there was not a bird or bunny to be seen. We still have no squirrels but we now have beautiful birds and precious hosta-eating bunnies. Mom will have to use that stinky spray again. All five of us are in our beds and ready for sleep.

We continue to monitor Steve King (boy, did Stephen Colbert give him a hard time or what!)

Sleep well, my friends!

More From March 21, 2017

We found out today that my cousin Boz had four seizures yesterday. They decided they could increase his dose of meds and that will work for a few days but it will be time soon to help him over the rainbow bridge. He played ball some on Sunday and enjoyed his time with family and had a slow day today. He's struggling to get his back legs uncrossed which is a result of the brain tumor interfering with motor signals. My auntie has already benefitted from your prayers for him and the love and support you've sent. It's going to be so very hard for them to let him go but she is stronger now than last week.

My folks, when they leave, always tell me that they'll be back and I hope when it's my turn to go over the rainbow bridge, they tell me they'll be back. All is peaceful here tonight and I spent an hour in the yard today! It was glorious lying in the sun! Even the cats are getting over Bella and ignoring her.

Mom and Dad have finally figured out my pattern of getting diarrhea. I get it whenever Bella and Bucket come or leave so now I get Pepcid and anti-diarrhea med at the first sign. Worked like a charm. Please remember, don't shop, adopt instead. There are so many of us who need homes. Praying good warm spring weather brings many pet adoptions.

March 23, 2017

Mom finally went to the doctor. She has bronchitis. Anyway, we had a very quiet day and Mom is NOT a good patient. She hates being still and sitting around feeling like a slug. This has been going on for three weeks and she says she sick and tired of being sick. So this will be short...as of this second unless, somewhere in this post, Mom changes her mind. We are saddened by the terrible killings in London. Mom and Dad say we get too comfortable with our everyday lives and become less and less aware. Mom read Gavin DeBecker's book, The Gift of Fear, and has re-read it twice. It says that (see, Mom is now not keeping it short) we become numb to that tiny voice inside our heads that says, "something's not right here" and we need to pay attention. That's how I got saved.... a policeman noticed me and noticed something wasn't right. So he saved me. He did the right thing. That's all we have to do is the next right thing. Bella and I reached a huge milestone captured below.

March 24, 2017

Observations of the day:

1. Vinegar with the Mother plus honey and lemon juice in warm ware is the best ever cough syrup.
2. The plus side of bronchitis is lack of appetite.
3. Sun on my back does feel really good.
4. Bella goes to the farthest corner of the yard to do her business and tries to be sneaky about it.
5. Being outside is stimulation for me and I love the smells and sounds.
6. I wobbled around pretty good today.
7. Buddy tries to hide all the toys in the dining room.
8. The best place to gnaw on the bone is under the bed.

Do something really special tomorrow and buy a bag of dog or cat food and just drop it off at the shelter nearest you. You will feel good and they will be thrilled.

March 24, 2017

We received this from my auntie this morning:

Sweet Bozzie crossed over the rainbow bridge this morning about 8:45. He is running and doing his flying lotus with Maggie. We think he had a stroke after I put him to bed. When I went at 1:30, he was on the blanket by my side and was not able to focus or move. We thought he was gone 3 x, but true to form, it was all on his terms. John came at 2:30 and once we realized he was breathing calmly, he went back home. I laid beside him all night just soothing him, although he was very restful. Taryn, Molly and Sue Murphy came at 8:30. Cameron and John were here. It was really hard for everyone, not a dry eye in the bedroom. Feels like a shotgun hit my gut. Weenie never left his side, even went under the bed by him. Pearl fretted until he passed, then became eerily calm.

So we ask for your healing energies to be sent to my Auntie's family. We trust that Boz is free to go on to his next journey full of health and perfection. We are all thankful he was able to die peacefully and not in the throes of a terrible seizure. The owner of Sycamore Veterinary Hospital in Midlothian, Virginia is Tarryn and the vet tech who kept Boz many times is Molly and the veterinarian is Sue Murphy. Boz's family and mine have been clients of this magnificent practice for over 30 years. We are all so grateful for their love and help.

We are also grateful for your prayers and support and know that this was a blessing in many ways,

March 25, 2017

Thank you all for the wonderful words and kind support to my auntie and her family. We have had a quiet day, and as you probably know too well, my mom has shed some tears. My auntie and my uncle are just trying to breathe and many of you know about experiencing this firsthand. We are really thankful that Bozzie went gently and peacefully and not suffering from a massive seizure or being unable to move around on his own. I did have my acupuncture this morning and I have done my best to fill the room with happiness. It occurred to me that none of us ever really own another creature's life. I don't own my parents' lives and they don't own mine. We are all only borrowed and blessed by the borrower.

March 26, 2017

We took a night off last night so we will catch you up tonight on our weekend. Bella and Bucket went home Friday night so we have had a quiet weekend. My anxiety at night has returned and even though I spent a good hour in the yard today, I've been whining a lot tonight. I really want to lie on my left side but it is painful for me to turn that way. Mom is going to see if maybe a muscle relaxer would help when she calls vet tomorrow. I'm just so tired of being on my right side.

It's also time for both Annie and Buddy to have their senior panels done at the vet so she has to call them anyway. Mom massaged me and brushed me but that didn't help. She put the heating pad under my blanket but I got too hot.

I have my favorite spot in the yard to do my business so now Mom and Dad have to re-sod because all the meds I'm on have killed the grass and made the soil awful. Any suggestions on correcting this will be appreciated.

Boz's family appreciates all the love sent to them by you. Thank you for the love and support you all shown for me and my whole family.

Please remember to microchip your pets. We see pictures of lost pets every day and wish so much people would microchip their fur babies. Many animal rescues sponsor discounted microchipping so if you haven't had yours done it is your turn!!!

March 29, 2017

We've been MIA for a couple of days but all is well. Mom has a very busy week next week with rehearsals and performances so we may miss some next week too. Mom has suddenly realized that she has geriatric pups (an oxymoron) with Annie being 11 and Buddy being around the same and me too. We are loving the sunshine and being outside when Mom is cleaning up the landscaping.

I'm not moving around much so Mom and Dad are trying to make sure I get to be in the sunshine when it is out. I have a very raw spot on my right hip from the hours and days I spend on my right side.

Mom and Dad are trying to make sure I don't drag myself around and break it open. So 1/2 of me is strong and 1/2 of me just won't cooperate. We keep hoping for a few more days of me wobbling in my own. We are thankful for today and for our freedom to enjoy it. We strive for wisdom in every day.

March 30, 2017

It never ceases to truly amaze me how your prayers and healing messages affect me. It is hard to put into words how this realization continues to wash over me. Today was a good day. I stood on my own, I needed very little help in the yard. I have been up to my water bowl on my own. We are amazed. We are thankful. We are grateful. My life continues to be filled with blessings. This day was a good one.

March 31, 2017

Somebody must have sprinkled happy dust over me last night while I slept! I slept until 9:00 this morning (and so did some other people I know) and have been happy all day. I've tried three times this evening to get Annie to play but she is not cooperating. I wobbled in the yard on my own so I am feeling better than two days ago. Mom and Dad found out that they can get my meds a lot cheaper at Costco and they are very happy about that!!!!!!!

Spring cleaning continues at our house and yard work will begin tomorrow if we don't have a bunch of rain.

We are sending our special prayers tonight to Trio Animal Foundation for the recent rescues that need many prayers. We trust that your prayers will include them.

Love to all!

April 3, 2017

Didn't mean to miss two posts in a row. We are a big football and basketball family so there has been some pre-occupation around here. I am about the same. No really bad days for almost a week so we are thankful!

Mom has an observation: in doing the spring cleaning and preparing for a yard sale, she has realized that all the wonderful heirloom China and silver and crystal are not things the 30-something people want. The gorgeous hardwood furniture of mahogany and walnut and cherry that was made right here in the USA has been replaced by the popularity of Crate and Barrel and Restoration Hardware. All stuff made in China, and stuff they can get rid of and change without a worry. It's so so sad. Mom's great-grandparents had some of our furniture and so did her grandparents. Every week, we see the little auction house up the road selling solid cherry dining room furniture...chairs someone paid $400-$700 each for now being auctioned off for nothing. She says the "throw away" generation will obliterate family things and along with it the family stories and history. She says you can hardly even sell Waterford crystal anymore.

Anyway, for hopefully many more years she will keep her China and crystal even if it does stay in the China press most of the time. By the way, I'm still eating out of a stainless steel bowl so she hasn't resorted to serving my meals on China every day.
Now, back to the game!

April 5, 2017

Dr. Ruth came today and I had a wonderful therapy session. I took a long nap afterwards and then enjoyed some time in the yard. Dr. Ruth worked on the muscles and nerve points in my back to keep the signals going to my legs. I love when she comes to see me and she spoils me with special treats every time. It's so cool that she has her own business now and comes to our house.

Mom had rehearsal tonight so we are all headed to see the sandman.

And! We have baby blue birds in our birdhouse! Yayyyyy. I will say special prayers of thanks for each of you.

April 8, 2017

Well, Mom has been at rehearsals every night since Tuesday and had the first performance tonight and the second one tomorrow night. She is singing the Britten War Requiem, and it is a grueling piece according to her account. There is no intermission, and it is a solid two hours! She says there are connoisseurs of Britten who love this work; however, she has yet to be persuaded. We have about been blown away today with winds whipping through here like it was March! It was also cold outside, so we didn't spend a long time in the yard.

As the world keeps on twirling, all of our household is praying for the wisdom our leaders need. Mom says that as a child she believed Peace would come to all of the world and now she knows that it probably won't happen in her lifetime but prays it will happen in the lifetime of my human sister. As for me, it usually takes me a couple of days after my acupuncture to get going again and I was slow today. But, I am just going to keep on keeping on. My silky back legs don't want to go where I need them to go. Dad and Mom step in and keep me from dragging myself. I'll take all the help I can get! So just for grins, here is a picture of my human sister's horse.

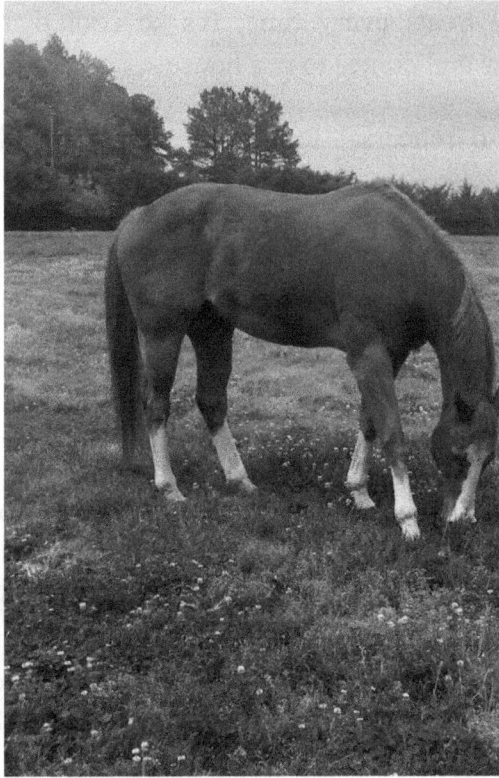

Head Over Heels, aka Leggz

April 9, 2017

Mom is finally home this evening. Poor Dad and us had to fend for ourselves every night this past week. Mom's rehearsals and performances were a brutal schedule. She sang with the Master Chorale with the North Carolina Symphony and they performed Britten's War Mass (Requiem). It is at this point the least favorite of the things she has sung. I stayed outdoors today for a good while when Dad was doing the edging and cleanup. I was quite up today and even tried to walk out the door by myself. It wasn't too successful but I sure tried. So we greeted Holy Week with beautiful azaleas and dogwood and lilac in full bloom. We pray your week will be peaceful and thoughtful and that you pass peace to others.

April 11, 2017

All is well. Busy day here and I loved being outdoors! More tomorrow! Thank you all for the blessings and prayers. The day was filled with bad news, so count every blessing and send all the healing light you can to those suffering parents in San Bernadino!

April 14, 2017

It's a busy weekend for all who celebrate the Christian Holy Week as well as the Jewish Seder. I want to be especially thankful for my Facebook Family and my ability to still enjoy this life. Blessings to all of you, and may hope be abundant in your lives.

April 17, 2017

We had a wonderful Easter Day and hope your day was as good. I had my time in the yard and got to watch the mommy and daddy bluebirds feed their babies in our birdhouse! We have beautiful cardinals and yellow finches every day now so all of the planting and feeding is paying off. Mom would be happy if she could remember what she planted and where last year, but she can't so now she just has to wait and see. The hosta are up and the Cala lily are too! But some of the green things she can't remember planting.

Buddy went on a run today. He's what Mom calls a "runner" and he slipped out of the garage door when they were working around the yard. He went two blocks away, and if he was smarter he would go between houses, but thankfully he stays on the sidewalk and is easy to spot. Now, Mom isn't saying he's dumb, but I don't think he's the brightest crayon in the box! But he surely is a momma's boy and we all love him to the moon and back.

Annie, however, got into the pantry when the door was left open, and ate an entire loaf of bread! She is now known as Miss Piggy and is on a diet. The only good dog was me!

My auntie's house is very empty without Boz and we think about him every day. Tonight we say a prayer for all those of you who have loved and lost a pet. We also pray that if you are able, you find your way to another pet who needs love and a home.

Today was all about hope. Hope for life, for forgiveness, and for wisdom to do good on this earth.

April 18, 2017

Needless to say, Annie is on a diet. She's just a piggy when it comes to food and Mom has to watch to make sure Dad doesn't slip her anything from his plate. Mom still can't believe Annie ate a whole loaf!

Buddy was NOT headed home when Mom found him yesterday. He was two blocks up the street walking towards the last street in the subdivision. I tried to tell Mom to give him credit for walking on the sidewalk, and not in the street, but she's not buying it yet.

It's been music madness in our house and it continues. Mom has rehearsals and performances every night this week beginning tomorrow through Sunday. They are singing Beethoven's Ninth (otherwise known as a soprano scream fest). So have no fears if my posts are sporadic! We will be back to normal after this marathon is over!

Life is good, we are blessed, and each of you is part of the reasons for this. Thank you.

April 19, 2017

Beethoven was deaf when he wrote the 9th. Mom says she's deaf when singing it. I'm sharing.

April 24, 2017

And the Beethoven marathon is over!! Mom is home tonight and actually cooked dinner for Dad. We all missed her and our schedules got slightly out of whack. She walked in the door this morning at 12:39 am just getting home from performing in Wilmington, North Carolina.

Now we have rain! We have rain and rain and rain. Our street is flooded and mom has to wear her boots to take me outdoors. Water is standing 2" deep in the yard because it can't soak up any more. Plants are loving it! Thanks to one of you I have a great raincoat so I don't mind so much. Here is the big news! When Mom was out in the yard with me on Saturday, she saw what she thought was one of our toys in the yard (Buddy loves to carry them out but NEVER brings them back in). It wasn't a toy! It was a beautiful wounded mourning dove who could not fly. Mom tried to get it but it hopped through the fence into our next door neighbor's yard. Mom decided to let it be and to check on it in an hour.

Well, an hour later it was still in the same spot. So, Mom got a sheet and went next door, covered the poor thing and scooped it up. We had a large deep box in the garage so Mom let it into the box, put birdseed in and a water dish. She covered it, left air holes, and........ it is still alive in our garage. She called wildlife rescue and sent pictures. She was told it is a fledgling and that it is trying to learn to fly, keep it in the box until the rain stops and then place it back in a safe place in the ground nearby. It is still raining and the poor bird is in the box, but safe and dry and warm. This event does not bode well for Mom vowing she would not take on anything else that needs her attention. She missed her calling. She should have run a rescue foundation beginning years ago! Annie, Buddy, Sandy, Lulu, Tipper, and now, at least for today we have Peace, the dove.

April 26, 2017

Good morning to you or to you who are still up... We had a busy day. My objective was to stay out of the way of rug machines and Dad touching up paint. It is indeed spring here. The sun finally came out around 1:00 pm! All the plants in the yard must have grown 6" because the rain made them shoot up! The grass needs cutting but the ground is still too soggy for me to even lie down on it. It was beautiful though to see the birds flocking to the feeder.

Our little Peace, the mourning dove, was set free today. Mom took the box out of the garage and Peace just walked out of it in a hurry. He was let out around our deck and some shrubs so Mom went back to check on him / her an hour later and there was no sign of it. It was in great health and tonight we will say a special prayer for the little dove, Peace.

Yes, Mom is a huge softie about creatures; except for spiders and fire ants and snakes. She won't be nursing any of those! My auntie's beach house took a big hit this past winter so Mom is going to the Outer Banks this weekend to help her get it ready for the rental season. Dad will be on duty!!! That means we will get fed late in the morning and early in the evening because he is a rack monster when Mom is away. He thinks she doesn't know it. Hahahah.

I am so thankful for social media and the way it has helped so many homeless animals. Awareness over the past 10 years has increased so much but there is still much to do. I sponsored someone to walk to raise money for the animal rescue here. His name is Fergus and his mom sings with my mom.

There are so many wonderful rescue stories out there. Maybe one day we can compile all of ours on my page!!

April 30, 2017

I plead guilty to taking a few days off. Mom headed to the Outer Banks to help her sister get the house ready for rental season and I proceeded to get a nice case of diarrhea. I get so upset if anything in my routine changes so now the chicken has been cooked and I will be getting rice and chicken only for a few days.

Mom has scrubbed and cleaned and is now collapsed on the sofa with both kitties wanting attention. Buddy goes in for his senior panel this week so please keep him in your prayers. Mom thinks he's going deaf but I think he has cocker spaniel selective hearing!

My auntie still misses Boz so much and she and my mom talked about how hard it is to lose a beloved fur baby. So tonight our prayers are for all of you who have a place in your heart that is empty because of loss. Perhaps the hole is meant to be filled in part by your next beloved pet and the loss becomes a blessed memory. Mom and Dad both have memories of their four-legged children.

I got my first dog when I was 7 years old. She was a blonde English Cocker Spaniel and I named her Tammy. I'd had a cat since I was a baby, and when Tammy came, my world was complete. Tammy lived until 1970, and died of a tumor on her lungs. I was so undone that I had to come home from school.

May 1, 2017

I think it's still March the way the wind is blowing. We even had to take in the rocking chairs from the front porch. There is some discussion about the big glass box and when it will be in use by me...... I need a nice dry warm sunny day so I can lie in the yard. It feels so good on my spine and legs.

As I write this, those silly cats are chasing each other through the house. They sound like a herd of elephants! Cats are weird.
So, happy it is May and I've lived a whole year and 3 months longer because of all the love and prayers sent my way!!!

May 3, 2017

Well, my mom's friend Anita came by today and I'll have you know that I got up and went to the kitchen to greet her!!!! She's very special and I really like her. Other than that I had a usual day and did get to lie in the bright warm sun!

So I decided tonight I'd tell you about our cat LULU. She was a feral kitten that was taken with her Mom and a sibling to a wonderful place that gives cats and kittens a second chance. Tipper had run away and been gone for a month so Mom couldn't stand not having a kitty... so she got Lulu. She is mostly Maine Coon but was a small kitten when Mom adopted her. One week later, Tipper came home. That's a story in itself for another day. So Mom and Dad have two cats. Lulu is not the sharpest tool in the shed. She is beautiful and hilarious but sometimes really bonkers. Now she weighs 13 pounds. It seems she has a problem with depth perception because she sticks her head under the faucet all the way to feel where the running water is, she uses her paw to feel the water if she drinks from a bowl on the floor. She jumps up to the bathroom counter whenever the water is turned on. She often misses.

Now, she either has a screw loose or she sees things we all don't see. She runs to the bathroom wall where the towels are hung and goes up underneath them and scratches the wall. If a door is left open to the closet or bathroom or master bedroom, she will close it and then proceed to scratch on it madly to get out. And, she can't see her treats if Mom puts them on the granite counter top in the butler's pantry. Mom tries to trim her nails and she turns into a ferocious tiger and will growl, spit and about claw you to death or bite you. So, Mom has the vet trim them and apply tips because Lulu thinks the oriental rug in the living room is her scratching post (by the way, she does have two of those but won't use them). She is extremely affectionate and thinks everyone who comes in the house is here to see her. To me she looks like an owl. Her purr is very loud and when she meows it sounds like a bird chirping. Tipper hates her but I think she's pretty cool...... who else has a cat that is half nuts and wags her tail like a dog. She's ok with me because she doesn't try to take my bed like some of the others around here.

Good night all and blessings on you.

May 5, 2017

Two big days in a row! Yesterday was Dr. Ruth and today was the big glass box. So I've been double relaxed and out like a light most of the day. My legs are significantly weaker and Dr. Ruth agreed with Mom and Dad that I have declined. I can't wobble much at all in the yard and so I just enjoy lying in the sun on the grass. My lower abdomen gets scalded and bad when I lie on my side so much with my legs together so Mom is propping my legs open with a rolled up towel. The bath today felt good and so did the medicine Mom used on me. I've not had my usual voracious appetite so Mom and Dad are watching carefully. This spinal thing is so cruel to take away my ability to walk and run when my brain still wants to. Please pass the word on genetic testing for DM prior to breeding for German Shepherds, Boxers, Corgis and all other dogs whose life is limited by DM.

May 9, 2017

Hello my good friends! This cool May weather is not my favorite so I'm going to be anxious for Sunday to get here and all the cool weather be gone. I'm really trying to still get up and get around. Occasionally now, I fall and can't get myself back up. My mind is so strong and my legs just won't work right. Mom and Dad get me up routinely to go outside and if Mom goes out of the room I drag myself into the bedroom to find her. The good news is that I still wait to go outside to do my business. We are all so thankful for that! I love getting hugs and being talked to!

My godmother Michelle sent Mom the sweetest Mother's Day card and it made her happy. We are thankful for this day and for my abilities to still enjoy life.

Don't forget to send your love to the mom in your life. And from me to all you moms of both two legged and four legged and some three legged babies, thank each of you for what you do, what you have done and what you will do for the babies you love who will always be your babies!

May 13, 2017

Wishing all of you moms of two legged and four legged children a wonderful day tomorrow. I know I am the mother of many German Shepherd pups and I have no idea where they are or if they survived but I do know I loved them and took wonderful care of them when they were mine. (If you ever got a GSD from Goldsboro North Carolina I might be their mom). I am happy now to have a mom who adores me, who hugs me and bathes me and makes sure I am well taken care of. I also have a wonderful Facebook Family and a wonderful woman who sends me monthly presents to help with all my medicine and acupuncture. She is a special person to do this for me!

Thank you from the bottom of my heart NH for being so constant. Moms are special people who will go without so their children will have, who bathe their children so patiently and lovingly, who clean up after us and go to great lengths to make sure we are safe and warm, never hungry or thirsty. It wouldn't be a world without moms and although my mom says I am a blessing on a daily basis, I know it works both ways.

May 15, 2017

I did go out in the yard this afternoon. It was a bit chilly today so not very warm in the sun. I am eating a little better. I still make it to my water bowl but cannot stand up to eat. I just give out. I now need help getting from my bed in the den to my bed in the bedroom. However, to Mom's surprise, I got up and made it to the toy box to get a ball. I'm getting lots of extra hugs and rubs and slept well last night. My meds keep me comfortable. For those who are new to my page please be assured that my mom and dad have me on every supplement they have found helps and I still get anti-anxiety meds to keep me from being so anxious at night.

Thank you my loving family for the prayers and the candles lit on my behalf. I will continue to try to fight and you inspire me on a daily basis. My mom and dad thank you too. They have never once lost patience with me, they help me to the yard every time, they love on me, and I feel very secure. What a nice feeling for an old GSD who lived most of her life being neglected and cold and mistreated.

My mom wishes to send her love and appreciation to all of you for the Mother's Day wishes. She hopes each of you celebrated in a way that made you happy and thankful. I may be weak in the hind legs but my appetite has not been affected at all! I do love my meal times!

Mom has begun putting her fingers in between the toe pads of my back legs. She hopes this keeps some of the nerve paths open that allow me to use them a little bit, and Dr. Ruth encouraged her to do it. I'm not so sure I like it very much but at least my legs still reflex a little bit. Dad made the comment today about how strong I am when I am ready to come back in the house and I pull on him. Mom told him that I wouldn't have survived this long without being willful and strong.

And so, today we are reminding ourselves that the glass is always half full and we are blessed in so very many ways. The God in us and with us is goodness and light and that is for us to share.

May 16, 2017

My auntie had to let Bozzie go over the rainbow bridge just three months ago. Today, she will let Pearl, her Southeast German Shepherd rescued GS go to meet him. She has a tumor that is in 70% of her lung and recurring cancer in a mammary gland. Please pray for Pearl's safe and comforting journey and for my Auntie and family as they help Pearl transition this afternoon. We pray that light and goodness and comfort and peace envelopes her and hope to see her again when we journey across the Rainbow Bridge.

May 18, 2017

Dr Ruth came yesterday so I slept most of the day after she left. Today, I must say, was a pretty good one. I was outside for a while in the shade and ate like a champ! I have amazed Dr. Ruth (she's really Dr. Ruth West, but I call her Dr. Ruth). She says she never expected me to be alive this long when she first saw me. Now, when she comes, I even get up and greet her sometimes. Getting up and down is a challenge and my back end doesn't cooperate very well but I still try and that's what is important. And, I'm still able to know when I need to go outside, and Mom and Dad are very thankful for that.

Thank you for the many prayers for my auntie and her family. Pearl was with auntie and my uncle as she transitioned and her bright spirit went to run and be with Boz and all of the wonderful creatures who have graced this earth. Each one of us, human or dog or cat or horse or bunny or living thing eventually must make the transition and so we must try harder to be kind and to love every day we have. Today was a good day. I breathed with ease, I saw the birds and the sky, I felt the warm sun and I had all the food and water I needed. I have a soft bed, a cozy home, and people who love me. I am blessed beyond measure.

May 22, 2017

It was a good weekend with steady keeping on. Mom says she notices me getting tired more easily. Getting up and lying down are very hard for me. It takes a good bit of cajoling to get me up even to put the harness under me. It may be time to put the Help Em Up Harness on me full time. I had a nice visit with Cash, the black Lab from next door and it really wore me out today.

Mom and Dad finished all the spring cleaning and yard so now Dad will be in charge of watering and Mom will do the daily vacuuming. Window sills all clean, paint touched up in whole house, bedspreads all clean, curtains dusted and fluffed, floors and carpets cleaned, grass re-sodded where I destroyed it (it was my favorite place to "go"), plantings done, shrubs pruned, trees fed, house power washed and windows cleaned. Whew!

Mom saw pets from a shelter today at Petsmart and loved on them. Don't forget to adopt not shop!!

Not a good day. I have been on my bed all day except when urged kindly to go out. I've had some accidents on my bed and thrown up three times in great volume. Will see vet tomorrow. Mom is tired.

May 23, 2017

It worked again!!! All your support and prayers and I am much better today. I ate chicken and rice and it stayed down and I don't have diarrhea anymore. It was a rapid improvement and just proves how the power of this loving family on FaceBook pulls me and my parents through over and over again! My dear Dr. Ruth texted my mom last night to check on me and have my mom check my tummy to see if I was bloated. I would not have the quality of life I have without her. She is my angel.

So because I am better please pray for the people of Manchester, for the young girls who will never graduate, for the fathers who won't ever walk a daughter down the aisle, for the mothers whose insides are torn apart, for the vigilant ones who sit beside hospital beds, for the nurses who tend them and wash them and medicate them, for the doctors whose skilled hands work to mend wounds, for the police who diligently work never ending hours to search and to secure, for the emergency workers whose lives will be ever changed by this tragedy. Pray for the evil to be wiped from the hearts of radicals, pray for our President as he journeys, pray for peace; peace in the hearts of the bereaved, peace in the minds of those in turmoil, peace for the souls departed.

May 28, 2017

And....... we have Bella and Bucket with us this weekend. Mom has figured out that I get my stomach in distress when Bella comes or when anything changes in my routine. I really am quite the worry wart and really want to be the Alpha dog with Bella but I can't keep up with her.

The Harness is helping a lot with getting me up and down. There's been a lot of laundry done this week due to my tummy but I am better. It's been nice for me to get outside, and Mom and Dad have a system now so they water the yard right after I try to kill the grass and it seems to help. I've also had several outdoor baths to get cleaned up but it is all working out.

Our good friends are moving to Florida this week and Mom and Dad will surely miss them. It will be lonely in the neighborhood without them.

Hope you have been able to fondly remember someone near and dear to you on this Memorial Day and that you count the sacrifices of so many on behalf of the USA as one of your blessings.

May 31, 2017

Our neighbors moved away today and Mom has been sad. Dad says Kevin was his only friend here, and Mom and I loved Anita's visits and the fun times. Mom says we live in a house full of seniors. Only the two cats are young, if young is 6 or 8. I was asleep earlier tonight and dreaming and Mom saw my back legs just running as hard as they could...... isn't that strange that when I'm lying down dreaming I can run but when I stand up I can hardly support my hind end at all.
Dr Ruth comes tomorrow!

Say a prayer tonight for the lonely dogs and kitties. And for the lonely people.

June 1, 2017

Dr Ruth came yesterday and I was so excited to see her that I had a hard time being still. I was wound up all day!!! When I am wound up I do a lot of whining and it worries Mom and Dad. So today around 2:00 I was really whining. So Mom and Dad took me outside and put me in my wheels. I wasn't very happy about it but I did walk up and down the alley about 50 feet which is a pretty big thing for me! Something very interesting happened when I was in my wheels. Mom and Dad noticed that I wasn't dragging either foot but moving them like I should. We can't figure it out...... I just cannot support my dear end but the dragging is less...??!! Mom will talk with Dr. Ruth about it tomorrow. I was exhausted after the short walk but we think it was good for me.

We can't believe it's almost been a year and a half since I was rescued. Who ever thought I'd be here this long? My loving Facebook family has been vital to my quality of life and we are all very grateful!

June 3, 2017

All is normal for us for the weekend. I've settled nicely into Bella and Bucket being here and my jealous nature has actually forced me to get up on my own several times to keep Bella away from Mom. My anxiety at night is increasing but I am eating well and bright eyed.
Our baby blue birds are about ready to learn to fly but we still watch Mom and Dad bluebirds feeding them in our birdhouse. The hummingbirds aren't here yet.

To the British and especially London, you are in our hearts

June 6, 2017

Bella and Bucket left Monday to go home to their mom. It is really quiet around here without them. Annie, Buddy and I are all finicky about going out in the rain so yesterday was no fun. Today was beautiful but I have been pretty low key. I slept a lot of the day and Mom brushed me. She says she got enough hair off of me to make another dog.

Mom is giving us all baths tomorrow if it is sunny. My auntie and uncle are coming this weekend to see us and I have to be all clean and fluffy. Buddy has to go to the vet because he has a funny cough when he lies down. Mom is taking precautions.

I have to have help most of the time now to get up but tomorrow we are going to go use the wheels for a few minutes to break the monotony. Here's to the sun coming up tomorrow and always hoping and praying each day will be a good one.

June 8, 2017

Today was good for all of us!!!! We all went to the dog park! Mom and Dad had the Harness on me and I walked around and sniffed the other dogs, sniffed and smelled the fresh air! Buddy is such a wanderer! There could be 50 dogs in there and he would still go off by himself wandering around like he's all by himself. He gets that from Dad. Annie, however, thinks everybody is there to see her and makes sure to socialize with every dog and every person. She gets that from Mom. Buddy's visit to the vet went well. She believes his tumors are truly fatty tumors, and he is slowing down a bit because he is a senior. All his blood work and stuff came back good so thankfully we don't have to worry about him. Last night when Mom took me out, Lulu slithered out of the door and vanished across the patio in a nano second. She has done this several times and there have been times when Mom is out looking for her past midnight. Mom wasn't in the mood to chase her so she just left her outside. Not to worry! In 10 minutes she was back at the door begging to get in. She really isn't right. At night she chases an unseen something through the hallway of the house and then tries to jump up the wall. See, I told you she isn't right!

Mom and Dad both celebrate birthdays today and the 10th so my auntie and uncle are coming for the weekend. I haven't seen them in a long long time. They were Bozzie and Pearl's mom and dad. We remind each of you shelters are so full in the spring and need towels and bath mats and blankets and bedspreads. They can use leashes and collars and flea and tick meds. So if you have time to drop off anything you think they could use, please do it! Baggies, rubber gloves, sponges and so many things!

Sandy does not cease to amaze us. She has such a sweet spirit and such a stubborn determination to be a part of everything. Both Annie and Buddy love her and she is even tolerant of Lulu and Tipper. Tipper actually goes to her and curls up against her to sleep.

We grapple each day to begin to face the inevitable deterioration that comes with DM. Sandy loves life, and for dogs with DM their minds are always willing but their bodies are unable.

June 10, 2017

Things I'm thankful for today that I spent most of my life not having:

Food
Bed
Clean Bed
Water
Fresh water

Saving Sandy   Diana B. Mahoney

Warm bath
Massage
Beautiful sunshine
My brother Buddy
My sister Annie
My kitties Tipper and Lulu
My Help Em Up Harness
My standing bowls
The yoga Matt in the floor
The special shampoo for my skin
My medicine and supplements
My collar
My blankets
My raincoat
My wheels
Being able to hold myself up
Being able to use my front legs
My eyes
My ears
My beautiful coat
Dr. Ruth
Lexi
GM Michelle
My Facebook Family
My mom and dad
My home
So many things and my family is blessed.

    And it's Dad's birthday!

June 11, 2017

Mom and Dad had my auntie and my uncle come to see us this weekend. My auntie loved on me and rubbed me a lot. She misses her Boz and Maggie and Pearl so much. She played ball with me and saw how much I have improved since over a year ago. She brought me all of Boz and Pearl's supplements and it surely is appreciated because my monthly meds and supplements are rather pricey. And, she also brought me and Annie the Adequan for Dr. Ruth to show my mom how to use. Mom and my human sister have used Adequan on our horse for years in his hocks and it made a huge difference. It may or may not help me but it can't hurt me. It is such a gift because it is sooooo expensive. If I didn't have good quality of life my mom wouldn't consider it but I do have a good life. A prayer of thanks for the wonderful things that have come my way!

What a surprise we got today from one of my Facebook family members! Special treats for me and special treats for my mom and dad!!! An unexpected joy! Just when you don't expect it, life drops a blessing on you. Don't miss it!!!!

June 14, 2027

How do I thank my sweet loving auntie for all the wonderful expensive medicine she saved that was Bozzie's and Pearl's.

Adequan has been used as an intramuscular injection for years with horses who suffer arthritic conditions and for a shorter time now with dogs. It is terribly expensive and there is only a possibility it will help me at all. But we are trying it and today I got my first injection. Dr. Ruth taught my mom how to inject when she came to do my electrotherapy and acupuncture. My mom has been routinely sticking her fingers into the middle of my toe pads to keep the nerve paths active. I jerk my legs back when I feel it. So today as soon as Dr. Ruth put the needle in my foot, my leg jumped so much it surprised her! That is a good thing! My mom and dad are feeling very blessed to be able to provide such goodness care to me. And in addition, one of my beloved Facebook friends sent Mom a box of special powder to keep the moisture away that comes from holding my hind legs together because I don't move them much at all.

So whether you are Republican, Democrat, or Independent, we need to all come together to recognize the value of life and that whatever we are doing to keep guns from people who shouldn't have them is NOT working. Mom says that doing the same thing over and over again and expecting a different result is the definition of stupidity.

Say prayers for the wounded people, the wounded animals in the world and for the stupid people because maybe it will help.

June 18, 2017

Dad is home with us this weekend because Mom went away for a long weekend with her college friends of 46 years! We've had terrible thunderstorms and I've been treated to boiled chicken and rice by Dad! I get all in a twist when Mom goes away and have diarrhea so Dad is sweet to fix the special food for me! I hope he knows that he's my security blanket when Mom isn't here and I love him. Mom comes home tomorrow so we will have Father's Day all together!
Happy Father's Day to all the wonderful dads out there.

June 19, 2017

Mom is home and recovering from relaxing. Dad took wonderful care of us and made sure we were ok throughout the thunderstorms.
I got my second shot today of the Adequan and we are all so hopeful it helps me. Annie is also getting it for her hips. Many thanks to NH

and GMM for what you have done for me and my lovely cards! Summer is settled in and we are blessed to have air conditioning and a comfy home.

One of the foundations that we support through Amazon Smile is Trio Animal Foundation. Miller is their therapy dog that helps acclimate the rescued dogs. He had surgery the other day and almost did not make it and still needs your prayers.

Please remember to use Amazon Smile when you order from Amazon. You can pick the charity or Foundation you want them to send money to. Even if you are a prime member, you can go to Amazon Smile and it recognizes you so you still get the free shipping with your order. We ordered our flea and tick stuff today because someone had a tick crawl up their arm after deadheading roses here in our yard. It wasn't me.

June 22, 2017

It's been a busy week!! Mom was home for a day then my parents had to make an overnight to see my dad's dentist. He had to have oral surgery to put a bone graft in his jaw so eventually he will have an implant whatever that is. He is now receiving lots of yummy soft food like mashed potatoes and pudding and Mac and cheese! PetnNanny took good care of us while they were gone but I'm just a piece of work. Mom hid her overnight bag from us, and did everything possible to keep us from thinking they were going away. But I knew! So, I promptly had diarrhea after they left and now I am perfectly fine.
I am due for my third Adequan shot tomorrow. So far, we don't see any notable difference but we are still hoping.

Trio's Miller was back in surgery today so we are hoping and praying he is ok.

June 23, 2017

Today I am officially a brat and Mom should have been a nurse. Got Dad up, poor Daddy, at 3 am, Mom up at 5am and again at 6 am, and I would not stop whining until Mom came to the den and slept on the sofa where my "your bed" is in the den. Never mind that I also have a bed in the master bedroom.

June 24, 2017

Well this is getting to be a habit. For the second night in a row I got Dad up at 3:00 am and Mom up at 7:00. I just lie in my bed and whine to wake Dad. Poor Dad is in pain still and not sleeping much at all. And I didn't help. I really did need to go out both times so Mom and Dad are looking at it as glass half full because I still recognize when I have to go out.

We may have seen a tiny wee bit of improvement in being able to stand up longer and get myself up a few times. My muscles in my hind quarters are wasting and they try to get me to walk around a bit in the yard but I don't much like it. I had a half bath today outside in the sunshine and I smell much better!

Good news about Miller and I know with all my heart that your prayers counted! Please continue to keep him in prayer and send all the healing energy you can to him.

June 25, 2017

Last night was a repeat. Dad up at 3, Mom up at 7. They even stopped my water intake early last night. Mom believes it's anxiety. Because if they wake up and talk to me and take me out I'm happy.

Mom says she's going to move my bed from in front of her dresser to beside her, but that puts me next to Buddy and we don't know how that will work out. Mom's almost ready to start sleeping in the floor with me. Almost but not quite. So apparently I had quite a few typos in my post yesterday and Dad noticed. So please excuse the fat paw pad.

A friend of Mom's has gone to work for the AKC. Interesting to find out the things they do for dogs who are not purebred or registered. It's good stuff!

Tomorrow when you wake up, think of me and smile at the next person you see. Tell them Sandy sent you!

June 27, 2017

I have a special request of my Facebook Family. I have emailed a request to the email below and ask you to email on my behalf to be considered for this test.

From Tufts University
Human patients could benefit from a study that's underway in dogs with a fatal paralytic disease
dog with wheels for support of back legs
"Giving these pets another one-and-a-half to two years of life would be a major success," Dominik Faissler said. "Better yet, we'd be doing something for dogs that at the same time contributes to human medicine." Photo: iStock
By Genevieve Rajewski
March 29, 2017

A gene-silencing therapy under development for people with amyotrophic lateral sclerosis (ALS) is being tested at Tufts in dogs with degenerative myelopathy, a fatal paralytic disease that is similar to ALS.

"If you look at the clinical progression [of degenerative myelopathy], a dog will go from dragging a toe, to stumbling, to falling over when it turns quickly," said Dominik Faissler, the veterinary neurologist at Cummings School who is leading the study. As the disease progresses, a dog can no longer stand.

"What's so extraordinary is that the dog is a naturally occurring model of one form of the human disease," said Robert H. Brown Jr., a University of Massachusetts Medical School neurologist who is one of the world's foremost experts on ALS and other neurodegenerative diseases. He approached Cummings School about testing the therapy developed in his lab, with the goal of speeding up clinical trials in humans.

"In dogs, it turns out there's a mutation in the SOD1 gene, which normally makes an antioxidant protein that helps protect nerve cells from a variety of cellular stresses and injuries. When this gene gets mutated, it becomes toxic to nerves, killing off the motor neurons in dogs the same way that this genetic mutation does in some people with ALS," said Brown, the Leo P. and Theresa M. LaChance Chair in Medical Research and chair of neurology at UMass Medical School.

Canine degenerative myelopathy causes progressive paralysis in older dogs in a number of breeds, including German shepherds, boxers, corgis, Chesapeake retrievers, Rhodesian ridgebacks and Bernese mountain dogs, Faissler said. "There is likely a genetic defect that interferes with the survival of the spinal cord tissue and brain tissue," he said. As in humans with ALS, dogs with degenerative myelopathy eventually die when the respiratory system stops working, but often pets are euthanized before.

The dogs in the Tufts trial receive a single spinal fluid injection of an engineered adenovirus—from a family of viruses that can infect the nervous system, but is best known for causing the common cold. The engineered virus was designed to breach the blood-brain barrier to deliver DNA particles that turn off—or silence—the mutated gene.

"This barrier is normally a very good thing, because it keeps bacteria out of our nervous system," Brown said. "But we must get the treatment to the cells where it can actually take effect, and a virus knows how to wend its way through that iron curtain." The therapy has shown promising results in mice genetically engineered to have a condition similar to ALS, he said, and it also was safe when tested in normal monkeys.

Dogs in the Cummings School trial, which began in December 2016, are checked every three months and undergo tests, which are videotaped, to assess their neurological and motor function. Four dogs are currently in the pilot study. So far, the therapy appears safe in pets, but Faissler and Brown said it's too early to determine whether it will halt or reverse the disease. "Does it work? That's the question I wake up and go to bed with every day," Brown said.

"Giving these pets another one-and-a-half to two years of life would be a major success," Faissler said. "Better yet, we'd be doing something for dogs that at the same time contributes to human medicine."

A successful trial in dogs could be a prelude to a clinical trial in people, Brown said. Ionis Pharmaceuticals, a California biotech company, is already testing a different gene therapy for SOD1-related ALS and for a similar type of mutation in patients with Huntington's disease, which attacks nerve cells in the brain. Such treatments one day could be used for a number of neurodegenerative and neuromuscular diseases, Brown said, including Parkinson's,

Alzheimer's and a host of diseases known as ataxias, characterized by the loss of control over bodily movements.

Veterinarians and pet owners interested in participating in the study should email neuro@tufts.edu or call Kellye St. John at 508-887-4839.

Genevieve Rajewski can be reached at genevieve.rajewski@tufts.edu.

June 27, 2017

Facebook Family: as requested, here is the email I sent to Tufts about being in the study on DM. Please look at my previous post to find the email address to send your email to. Thank you from my heart!

Hello,

My name is Sandy and you can see my daily chronicle on Facebook about my DM. Saving Sandy is my Facebook page and I have over 15,000 followers.

I am a rescued full German Shepherd. My foster failure parents have devoted their lives to me 24/7 for a year and a half. I have lost the ability to walk without losing control of my hind end, I am still strong in the front legs and eat well.

My parents have spent $10,000 in therapy and medicines to keep me comfortable and happy. We have documentation of all the things we have tried and are now on our 4th shot of Adequan just praying it will improve something.

I would be so honored to be selected for your program and my veterinarians would help monitor all behavior and changes. I receive acupuncture every two weeks. We have tried physical therapy, hydro therapy, and acupuncture. We continue acupuncture to give me some relief from the extreme anxiety I have from not being able to get around. I really don't want to lose my front legs too. Please consider me. My parents are retired and extremely dedicated to my well-being as well as the well-being of my brother and sister who are both rescued.

Thank you kindly,
Sandy Mahoney
(Much loved GSD of Diana and Michael Mahoney)

Diana B. Mahoney

June 28, 2017

I want to thank each of you who emailed on my behalf. It really got their response to us quickly. I have now written to them to tell them I can still walk. Not well, but I am able to get to my water bowl and my bed and support myself to urinate. I can't do steps.
Hoping they will reconsider: Here is the response I received early today.

Dear Mr. and Mrs. Mahoney,

Thank you for your inquiry into this clinical trial. I tried calling the number below to speak with you in person but I could not leave a voice mail. I'm sorry to tell you that Sandy is not eligible for this clinical trial due to the fact that she no longer can use her hind legs. This trial is designed for dogs that are still able to walk. We are trying to determine if this new treatment will halt or slow down the progression of this disease, and to be able to determine this, we need the dogs to still be able to walk when enrolled. As much as we would like to be able to enroll all dogs, we are not able to do this. This treatment is not a proven thing - that is what we are trying to determine. And in order to be able to determine if this treatment is beneficial, we need to establish a starting point and an endpoint. The starting point is dogs that have the double positive mutation on the SOD1 gene and are in the early stages of the disease and still able to walk. The endpoint of this is the loss of motor function to the back legs. As this is the way the science is set up, we are unable to enroll dogs that have already reached the end point. I hope you understand this. If you have any further questions regarding this clinical trial, I am more than happy to speak with you to answer them.

Kind regards,
Diane Welsh
Diane M Welsh, CVT
Clinical Trials Coordinator

https://vetinside.tufts.edu/wp-content/uploads/2016/03/Cummings-tagline-bw.png

200 Westboro Rd
N Grafton, MA 01536
508-839-5395 X84441
Fax 508-839-7922

Clinical Trials

Updated Jun 28, 2017, 12:52:08pm

June 28, 2017, continued

Facebook Family. After letting the Tufts Veterinary clinical Study coordinator know that Sandy can still walk, and calling the coordinator (I had to leave a message), we received this information.

Dear Diana,

I did not go into the full screening requirements in the previous email as I thought Sandy was no longer ambulatory. This study involves an injection following an MRI and CSF tap. This is followed up at 1 month with another CSF tap and then every 3 months, there is another recheck until the dog can no longer walk. All of these visits need to occur at our facility in North Grafton, Massachusetts. At all of these rechecks, there is blood work drawn and the dog is also walked across a force plate to evaluate the quality of their gait.

The inclusion criteria for this study includes having genetic testing showing they are affected by the SOD1 gene and an MRI proving that they do not have any other spinal cord diseases and recent normal chest x-rays and routine bloodwork. The dogs also still need to be able to walk on their own and weigh more than 30 pounds. We are looking for dogs in the early stages of the disease that are still able to walk.

If you feel that your dog may qualify, the next step is to make an appointment with our neurology service. If genetic testing has not been done yet, we can submit this at that time. The initial work up (genetic testing, MRI, neurologic exam) is not covered by the study. Once eligibility is determined and the owner consents to the study, then all medical expenses associated with the trial are covered. (Travel expenses are not covered)

This trial is currently on a hold for enrollment as the investigators did an interim analysis of the first set of dogs enrolled and found that we had not made any changes in the progression of the disease, and therefore, they are reformulating the injection that is to be administered. We are hoping that enrollment will be able to begin again in August, but we do not have a definite date.

As mentioned earlier, all study visits must occur here in Massachusetts. Some of the screening tests can be done at local veterinarians, with results forwarded here. Has Sandy had the genetic testing done yet? That would be the first test I would recommend having done if you are considering this trial and can make it to Massachusetts for all time points in the study.

The ultimate decision of eligibility will still require an appointment here with our neurologist so that each dog is examined and all the intricacies of the study can be discussed. I have concern as to whether or not Sandy's ambulatory ability is strong enough to be eligible. This is a hard thing to determine through email. I also have concern that since we are not able to enroll until August that she may not qualify at that time.

If you have further questions, I would be happy to talk with you tomorrow. I apologize for not getting back to you sooner, I had a crazy busy day and was not able to get to my desk till now.

Kind regards,
Diane Welsh

Clinical Trials Coordinator
508-887-4441
Fax 508-839-7922
clinicaltrials@tufts.edu

So, making 3 or 4 monthly trips to Massachusetts is a bit overwhelming for Mom and Dad since travel expenses are not included in the study AND, having the genetic test and MRI here at home would be out of pocket for Mom and Dad. Mom will call North Carolina State Univ vet School tomorrow to find out what that expense would be. Then Mom and Dad will talk. Mom is concerned that the stress on me would be more damaging in making the trip.

Later June 28, 2017

My mom and dad have decided that since I never knew peace and security until I came here, it is best that we not undertake a clinical trial that would make me have anxiety and fear. The 14-hour trips would mean I had to lie in the car for a half a day there and back even if I was approved for the study. I am happy and comfortable and content so they will continue to love me and nurture me right here at home for as long as possible.

I do want to tell you that the vet school reached out to Mom so fast and we know it was because of all your emails! This is ONE POWERFUL FACEBOOK FAMILY! We are in awe of the awareness that our posts create and thrilled that the veterinary school clearly knows how important DM research is to so many people. Thank you for being so loyal, so devoted and so generous with your time and hearts.

June 30, 2017

So....... although we try not to be too graphic about my health, it truly is a monumental day when I can again stand to go to the bathroom! Alone! Without falling! We are thankful and not asking how or why. I walked, not well, but walked around the yard yesterday and today! So for today that is enough.

July 3, 2017

Oh the ups and downs of this journey! I had a lousy day today. Did not want to eat breakfast and ate a very little dinner. Energy level was way down. So I'm off to sleep and maybe things will be better tomorrow.

Please, please remember to keep your pets out of this heat and make sure they have plenty of water. Don't ever leave your pet in the car in weather like this!!!

July 4, 2017

Mom says to tell all of you that Best Friends, the animal sanctuary in Utah, publishes a quarterly magazine and featured an article on DM! Morning feeding: I got Mom out of bed, went outside and did my routine. Came in, got on my "your bed." Mom fixed my breakfast and sat down to feed me. I turned my head. She turned my whole body to face her and presented me with another fork full. I turned my head. She held yet another fork full in front of me which I slowly took off of the fork and promptly dropped on my feeding mat. Mom got up and put the food away.

Dad had more luck at dinner because I was hungry. After dinner I actually caught the tennis ball 10 times. Sometimes if Annie or Buddy lie in front of the water bowl I whine and have a hissy fit. I do not like it when Mom has private conversations with Annie or Buddy so I interject my large self into the chit chat.

Wishing we could take a trip to the beach and I could use my wheels in the sand. It's been so blasted hot here. Dreading the fireworks tomorrow night. Mom will move Alexa into the master closet with us to play us soft classical music.

July 6, 2017

We survived the 4th with very few fireworks thanks to a long severe thunderstorm! Yayyyyy! Then Mom and Dad had to travel overnight to go see Dad's dentist to have sutures removed and now we are all back at home and settled. Of course, Annie, Buddy, Tipper, Lulu, and I stayed at home and had our wonderful PetnNanny come care for us.

Everyone always does fine when Mom and Dad are away except me. I refused to eat a bite and all I would do was take my meds with peanut butter. It causes Mom and Dad concern but they did preemptive Imodium before leaving so at least there wasn't that problem. I ate like a champ tonight and am lying at their feet feeling much better. My hind end has gotten really thin so Mom and Dad are faced with me not eating and what that means whenever they travel. (Which isn't much!)

House is wonderfully cool and outside is dreadfully hot. Hoping water is available to all the strays that are wandering hoping to be rescued.

July 9, 2017

We have finished our two per week shots of Adequan and now go to one a month. It has helped Annie significantly but has only slightly helped me. I have gotten pretty weak in my hind end and so if I can get up on my own I usually just stand in one place now until Mom or Dad comes to help me. We had hoped I'd bounce back a little more but we will take what we have and do our best with it. My days are beginning to consist of just lying on my bed and sleeping but Mom still tries to get me excited about going outside. I have eaten better today so maybe tomorrow I'll have more energy. Mom and Dad worry that this decline will soon take away my ability to even stand.

Yesterday was a classic Sandy day. I refused to eat my normal food so Dad cut up some cooked hot dogs and stirred them into my food. They tried that again this morning to encourage me to eat more, but true to my breed, I sniffed out those hot dog morsels and spit everything else out. I think they are on to me now.

Please remember that our paw pads burn on the hot pavement and we get dehydrated really fast in this hot weather! Tip for traveling:

freeze two bottles of water that will melt along the way and still be cold and travel with a water bowl!

July 10, 2017

Just a quick update. I am back to eating my normal amounts as of today. I am still able to let Mom and Dad know when I need to go out. I am still going to my water bowl but with great effort. I don't like to drink when I'm lying down so every time Mom brings the bowl to me I stand up so they are just letting me do it on my own as much as possible. Dr. Ruth comes tomorrow so I'll feel good tomorrow afternoon and probably sleep.

One of my Facebook family members did contact the owners of the GSD who won the dog show. They politely declined and we are thankful for the effort it took to contact them!

Mom has a friend who has started doing some work for the American Kennel Club so Mom is going to spend some time on their website to read about what they do.

Just think....... if research could come up with a cure for DM, there would be a path to cure Lou Gehrig's disease!

July 13, 2017

Dr. Ruth West came to give me my acupuncture and I loved it. I slept most of the day afterwards and yesterday had a pretty good day. I ate well and did ok getting to the yard and back. Today I slept late which Dad was thankful for. I am very alert when I am awake and have needed some help today getting to my water bowl. I've gotten really good about sniffing out the pills in my food and turn my head when I don't like what is on the fork. I am one smart cookie! It was the hottest day of summer so far here in North Carolina so I didn't get the bath outside because it was tooooo hot. Maybe tomorrow. My friend Dottie had to say her "goodbye for now" to her fur baby. We know he will be reunited with her and send her our love and prayers for her broken heart. We have a neighbor who found a lost dog yesterday and spent two hours driving and waiting for her owner to come home! She is a hero! The dog was six or seven miles from home. Blessed are those who rescue!

July 16, 2017

So we were checking today and somehow a post from Friday didn't post: (I had a really bad Friday and Saturday and wasn't able to use my back legs at all on Friday. We were all a bit alarmed and coming to terms with it. Then, this morning, I got up and woke Mom so I could go out, I ate a full breakfast and held myself up when I went outside this afternoon. It is a pretty good day! I've gotten lots of belly rubs and if it's not 90 degrees or higher tomorrow I'll get a bath outside! Our family is ever mindful that I won't ever be cured or able to run again but we are all grateful for me still being able to get up, to eat, and to be continent. We also know that I wouldn't be here in this ride if it weren't for the power of prayer and love. My heart is thankful for each of you. I'm lying here on my "your bed" in a comfy air conditioned home with no worries about my next meal or my safety. What more could anyone ask?

July 18, 2017

I am back to my normal and we are happy about it! My mom and dad are thankful for the patience that has been granted to them through the healing prayers and energies sent our way. Who would have ever imagined I would even be alive a year and 5 months from being rescued. Even Dr. Ruth West of Karma K9 Mobile Acupuncture says she would not have imagined I would do this well for so long. It is a miracle so to those who doubt that miracles happen, take a look at me. When Mom's patience is running out, Dad calmly steps in and Mom truly thinks of each of you and draws on your love for me to take a deep breath and restore calm to her being. Dad is always so calm and steady while Mom is the busy bee, always multi-tasking and forgetting why she opened the refrigerator or walked into the laundry room. Ha, don't even mention losing her glasses. She only has about 5 pair and manages to lose all of them.

Anyway, today we are thankful for the birds that come to feed at the feeder; cardinals, finches, wrens, sparrows, doves. And, we are thankful for the butterflies and precious hummingbirds that enliven our back yard. It reminds us of the lilies that neither toil nor spin........

July 21, 2017

I went to the vet today and had my nails trimmed. All of us had our nails trimmed except Tipper because she lets Mom do it. Lulu becomes a wild tiger and Mom doesn't even try anymore with her. The concerning news is that I've lost about 15 pounds. We knew I was losing weight due to the almost total loss of use of my back legs....... but we are increasing my meals and considering some other supplements. We also know that my being able to walk at all for this amount of time is a miracle and we are grateful for the time my legs have worked. Thinking about the progression of this awful spinal disease means my front legs are having to do double work and my shoulders are tense and tired. It's hard for me to walk, and I never walk but three or four steps without help.

I guess what I'm trying to say is that we all know this won't get better except for moments here and there. In fact, we know it will get worse. Mom and Dad will be with me all the way, and we hope all of you can begin to know that as I get worse, and when I tell Mom and Dad I've had enough, they will hold me up and carry me until I get across the Rainbow Bridge where I will run and jump and wag my tail forever.

Until then, we will be strong and we will be conscious of what is right and good for me.

Love to all,
Sandy

It was a welcome sight to see Dr. Ruth! I needed that treatment today so much! Mom and Dad talked with her about my decline and she was in agreement that I've lost more of my muscle and ability to walk. We talked about what to expect and what to look for in the days to come. I do feel less stressed tonight after the acupuncture and enjoyed a nice dinner of chicken and rice after refusing to eat my breakfast. I am not in pain. The only thing that ever hurts is if I fall too hard or if I get too far over to my left. The anxiety about not being active and being able to go where I want to go is the worst thing. Sometimes my stomach gets upset but Mom and Dad know just what to do for that. So here is my deep appreciation to all of you and a special thank you to all the parents of disabled dogs who work 24/7 trying to make sure we have quality of life. And extreme compassion and appreciation to those who walk the journey to the end of our earthly life.

I have found that dousing a cotton tip in pure Lavender oil helps to calm Sandy, so it is a nightly ritual. Her poor shoulders and front legs are so sore, and the acupuncture helps so much. I only wish I could take away her pain.

July 26, 2017

So today's post is not about me. My mom wants to post something she posted on her own Facebook page, because she feels it's important.

I'm sorry...... I cannot help but be sick at heart and now doubtful about the integrity of anyone who would vote to put this thug into the Hall of Fame. I have held his wounded and scarred dogs in my arms. I have fed them and sat on a concrete floor waiting and waiting for one to trust me enough to crawl on her belly across the floor to me. She had no teeth. She was a breeding female whose teeth had been pulled so she would not bite a male on the rape stand. This thug is infamous and only deserves to spend his time in service to an animal support organization.

NEW RIVER VALLEY
Virginia Tech Veterinary College dean releases statement against Vick Hall of Fame induction
By Jeff Williamson - Digital Content Manager
Posted: 3:19 PM, July 24, 2017
Updated: 1:42 PM, July 25, 2017
29 Comments
Michael Vick is one of five athletes being inducted to the Virginia Tech Sports Hall of Fame.
BLACKSBURG, Va. - Not everyone at Virginia Tech is in agreement about Michael Vick being added to the Virginia Tech Sports Hall of Fame.

The dean of the university's College of Veterinary Medicine said in a statement, "The College unequivocally opposes honoring an individual whose past actions contradict our values and the cornerstone of our mission."

More New River Valley Headlines
Virginia Tech facing criticism for Michael Vick Hall of Fame induction.

The university made the announcement on July 11 that the former quarterback would be honored.

Vick, who finished third in the 1999 Heisman Trophy voting – the top finish ever by a Tech player – went on to become the No. 1 overall pick in the 2001 NFL Draft.

Vick was a quarterback for the Atlanta Falcons in 2007 when his life off the field drew national attention. Vick and three other men were indicted on charges related to a dog-fighting ring known as "Bad Newz Kennels." His involvement and subsequent prison sentence have made him a controversial figure in sports.

Vick, and the other four new honorees, will be inducted during a Hall of Fame dinner on the Tech campus on Friday, Sept. 22, the evening before Tech's home football game against Old Dominion. The inductees will then be introduced to fans at halftime of the football game.

Read the complete statement from Virginia-Maryland College of Veterinary Medicine Dean Dr. Cyril Clarke:

The recent decision to induct Michael Vick into the VT Sports Hall of Fame has generated a tremendous response from both the veterinary community and those who share our commitment to animal welfare and promoting the humane treatment of animals. The Virginia-Maryland College of Veterinary Medicine was not part of the nomination process nor the decision, which was made by a committee of past athletes. The College unequivocally opposes honoring an individual whose past actions contradict our values and the cornerstone of our mission. Over the course of several days, I have communicated with President Sands and other campus administrators to express our disappointment and opposition to this decision. I continue to be in conversations with the president regarding this issue. The College of Veterinary Medicine will continue to stand behind our mission and advocate for an alternative outcome. Our mission has not changed and we will continue to work tirelessly to advance programs that promote the welfare of animals and be a strong voice that reflects our unified commitment to compassionate care and our dedication and respect for the animal lives that benefit from the education and care we deliver.

IF YOU SHARE MY MOM'S OPINION, PLEASE WRITE TO THE PRESIDENT OF VIRGINIA TECH AND REMEMBER TO PASS IT ON!

Thank you so much. We are from Virginia and feel this man is an embarrassment and that this recognition sends the wrong message to our children!!

July 27, 2017

Please go to change.org and search for petition to keep Michael Vick from being inducted into Virginia Tech Hall of Fame https://www.change.org/p/president-tim-sands-stop-virginia-tech-from-inducting-michael-vick-into-the-sports-hall-of-fame

It's working! My mom does not try to promote causes on my page but she's passionate about this one because of her up close and personal experience with the victims. She doesn't mean to offend anyone but truly believes this a poor example for our children, for students at the college and does not believe he paid the dues because no one can do the things he did who has any respect for people or animals. Please sign the petition, and email the governor of Virginia, the president of the college. There is no time to spare.

Stop Virginia Tech from inducting Michael Vick into the Sports Hall of Fame. Jennifer Breeden Warrenton, VA 61,537 Supporters I am a Hokie. I have always been proud to be a Virginia Tech alumni until the University recently announced its decision to induct Michael Vick into the VT Sports Hall of Fame. I am also an avid animal lover, particularly dogs. In 2007, Michael Vick pled guilty for his involvement in a dog fighting ring and spent 23 months in federal prison. Along with abuse, torture and execution of dogs, drugs and gambling were involved. If you are a dog lover and advocate, a sports fan, a Hokie or none of the above, you've probably heard the gruesome details about this case.

By inducting Michael Vick, a non-graduate, into the Virginia Tech Sports Hall of Fame, the University has decided to honor a man for his athletic ability rather than honor a person for being a decent and honorable human being. I would hope a top leading University, especially one who has an excellent Veterinary Program, would take a second look at themselves and evaluate what they want to be known for. Michael Vick should be anything but honored at Virginia Tech, and absolutely not inducted into the VT Sports Hall of Fame. This petition will be delivered to: Virginia Tech President Tim Sands. Read the letter Jennifer Breeden started this petition with a single signature, and now has 61,537 supporters. Start a petition today to change something you care about. Start a petition.

Please go to change.org and search for petition to keep Michael Vick from being inducted into Virginia Tech Hall of Fame

https://www.change.org/p/president-tim-sands-stop-virginia-tech-from-inducting-michael-vick-into-the-sports-hall-of-fame

July 28, 2017

Please continue to read posts below to sign petition!

On another topic, we found this today! We think maybe you'd like to read this:

Canine Degenerative Myelopathy Test Moves Toward Trial
Researchers from the University of Missouri are looking for dogs for
the clinical trial.

BY VETERINARY PRACTICE NEWS EDITORS
Published: 2017.07.27 05:55 AM

Similarities between dogs and people are well studied, so it's unsurprising that researchers discovered a test used to diagnose amyotrophic lateral sclerosis (ALS) in people is applicable to identifying degenerative myelopathy (DM) in dogs.

The genetic link between the diseases was established in 2009 by Joan Coates, DVM, Dipl. ACVIM, a professor at the University of Missouri (MU) Department of Veterinary Medicine and Surgery, and other researchers at the Broad Institute at MIT and Harvard.

While the current genetic test for DM can identify risk for the disease, it's limited in its ability to diagnose it. Therein lies the problem, because as of now, a proper DM diagnosis is time-consuming and expensive, requiring procedures such as MRIs of the spinal cord, according to Dr. Coates.

"DM is a diagnosis of exclusion, meaning that veterinarians must rule out all other diseases that mimic it before coming to a final diagnosis," Coates said. "Now that we know that DM and ALS are related, we are studying ways to diagnose and measure disease progression with similar diagnostic modalities used in ALS patients."

Coates and her MU colleagues have developed a simple DM diagnostic test based on a similar one used to diagnose ALS in humans. Specifically, they found elevated levels of phosphorylated neurofilament heavy proteins (pNF-H) in the cerebrospinal fluid and blood samples—the same biomarkers appear in humans with ALS— of dogs with DM compared to dogs without it.

"These results will enable us to 'scale up' the test to make it more accessible to [the] veterinary community," Coates said. "pNF-H may serve as a diagnostic tool for diagnosis of DM."

With the link between ALS and DM established and a new test making diagnosis easier, now Coates and her team are seeking pets to take part in a clinical research trial into treatments for DM that slow its progression and improve the patient's quality of life.

The MU research team is collaborating with other ALS scientists, and the studies are being funded by the ALS Association and National Institutes of Health.

"Dogs suffer from more than 350 genetic disorders, many of which resemble human conditions," said Ewen Kirkness, Ph.D., a molecular biologist at the Institute for Genomic Research, now the J. Craig Venter Institute, in Rockville, Md. "The genes responsible for these are probably constant to humans and dogs."

The research by Coates and others shows that benefits can be derived by taking a closer look at these links.

"I was very excited by the idea that there could be another model that might have more strength than the existing models," said Michael Garcia, Ph.D., an assistant biology professor and principal investigator at the MU Bond Life Sciences Center, who is working with Coates on the research, about the new DM diagnostic test.

The DM treatment trial will occur at the MU Veterinary Health

Center Small Animal Hospital; dog owners interested in their pet participating can email coatesj@missouri.edu.

July 29, 2017

I am happy that today is cooler but boy, did we have a thunder boomer last night! Mom is exercising my legs and sticking her fingers between my toes to try to help the nerve pathways stay active. We've emailed the people about the DM study and hopefully will hear back next week. I haven't had my usual appetite but I ate a big dinner tonight.

Now, I have to tell you a story: Mom saw on Facebook that there was a couple in the county close to my auntie in Virginia who had a rescued German Shepherd about 5 years old. My auntie hopped right on it by using some of her dog contacts and the dog was found in the county over from where my auntie lives; she had ticks all over her and was in very poor condition and starving. Some kind people had taken her in when they found her crawling up their driveway. They bathed her and got rid of ticks but they have 3 dogs and knew this dog needed more space and medical attention so they turned to the shelter. The shelter took her to be examined.

The long and short is that she has Lyme disease and elbow dysplasia. She also has a mammary tumor. My auntie is working hard to find out how to get the right treatment, if possible, for this girl who is only about 5 years old. So we have encouraged her to set up a GoFund Me account for her if possible and if treatment is a viable option. Her name is Sally and you won't believe this! The man and woman who found her and fed her and bathed her used to work with my mom and my auntie! This is a miracle in itself!!
I will be keeping all of you posted on Sally.

P.S. I have learned that whining loudly when I want to get up works very well.

July 31, 2017

We have had a bad couple of days. I am unable to get up by myself for the second day in a row. Dr. Ruth comes tomorrow so we will be evaluating me. I no longer go to my water bowl without help. It's frustrating and makes me whine a lot.

August 1, 2017

Mom had her days wrong. Dr. Ruth comes tomorrow. I had a nice bath outdoors today and lay in the sunshine to dry off. Dad held me over his knees while Mom scrubbed. All the activity wore me out and I'm on my "your bed" covered up so I don't get chilled. I ate a good dinner. I'm so lucky my dad is so strong! He carried me to the blanket to lie in the sunshine.

August 2, 2017

My mom and dad and Dr. Ruth are all on the same page. I have begun to swing my front legs to the side when I am up being helped to walk. My shoulders are sore and tired. So I'm getting the royal treatment with lots of being waited on and loads of hugs and little chats.

I can't squat at all anymore to use the bathroom so Mom and Dad are helping with that. I have good meds for my anxiety and discomfort.

I know that all your prayers and love are what has made my life so full and each one of you is special to us. This journey is the journey home, where I will walk again and run and be able to wag my tale. We are looking forward to the next week for me to be spoiled and comforted and loved. Pray for my mom and dad ......they are trying to be so strong for me.

Our next week will be a trip to the lake, lots of yummy food, and lovely time in the sun. Cool drinks of water, bones and massages.

August 3, 2017

We are making the most of every precious day. Yesterday was really hard on Mom and Dad. Heartfelt thanks to everyone who sent love and prayers. You will be their strength in the coming days.

I have stopped being able to walk, and my bladder control is waning. I'm not having a really good time anymore. So we will spend the next week of my life doing special things in preparation for my last earthly journey.

..... special marrow bone!

..... special marrow bone!

A marrow bone!!!! Yummy!

August 5, 2017

At the lake in the shade! Beautiful day and I've loved sniffing the air and the pine needles!

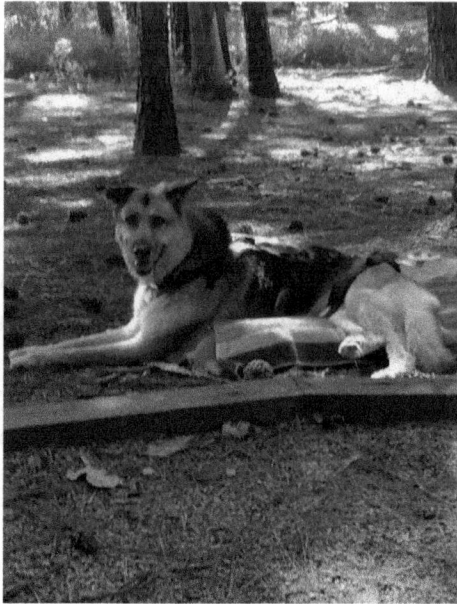

August 6, 2017

My mom and dad want you to know that they do read your posts. It is just that they have to do it slowly right now. Thank you all for everything you have done for us. I am eating well and being pampered. I'm getting Boar's Head turkey and turkey hot dogs and frozen marrow bones. I am being assisted to the yard and I get to wander and stand as long as I care to.

Mom keeps looking for a sign that I am better and clinging to any little thing, and then she has to remind herself that it is quality of life that matters not quantity.

Mom will talk with Dr. Thames tomorrow. I'm not in pain, just tired and frustrated. I am still getting my meds and Annie is keeping a close eye. Here's to tomorrow and thankful for today.

This sucks. This hurts. My heart is breaking. How can I let her go? She has been my life for a year and half. She deserved to live and be happy for a long time. I tried too hard to accept that this journey would not end well.

Later in the day, August 6, 2017

We would like to know where each member of my Facebook family lives. That book Mom talked about a year ago may get written and we want to include all the names and places of her family. So if you'd be kind enough to just post your state or country we'd like to keep a record of it and use it in a helpful way to tell Sandy's story to the world. What a family we have become. A family of strength and love, compassion and unselfish act of kindness. It's a remarkable story about remarkable people saving a remarkable dog.
Thanks for sharing with us.

August 7, later in the day

Mom hasn't been very good about acknowledging every comment yet because she says her eyes won't stop leaking. I am spending my days on my "your bed" getting special food and lots and lots of love.

From Mom: We are so grateful for all of your love and support. We are doing everything we can to make this a special comfortable week. Sandy is a gift and we will always be thankful for the patience she taught us and the love she shared with us. Her return to her eternal home and unbounded energy will be a gift of freedom we can give her at the end of the week.

August 10, 2017

I had a special trip to McDonalds today. I got two hamburgers and was really happy! And tonight Mom actually let me have some of the kitties' treats. Mom has said she is planning to gather all my posts and put it into a book so maybe it will help other abused and neglected dogs find homes.

My auntie did adopt the badly neglected German Shepherd that I told you about last week. She has to have surgery on mammary tumors and has terrible shoulder issues. Her name is Gabrielle and they call her Gabby. The shelter was calling her something else so it will take her some time to get used to her new name. We received many good wishes today and a lot of love. We thank you and ask you to pay it forward in honor of me and my journey.

Love Sandy

Later August 10

As some of you know, my auntie lost her three German Shepherd dogs within a year and a half. Last week, she rescued a neglected German Shepherd who has shoulder dysplasia but who is a young dog with a wonderful loving personality. She needs to be spayed and have some mammary tumors removed. Her name is Gabby and she looks like me. Mom and Dad are praying for strength and courage as they carry me to the Rainbow Bridge tomorrow. It is very hard for them as for so many of you know and anyone who is brave enough to put their pet's comfort before their own need to keep the ailing pet alive. We are thankful for your love and your kindness to us.

Hold us tightly in your heart as we travel along this journey to my health and wholeness. Celebrate tonight by squeezing your fur babies extra tightly and look into their eyes and tell them you love them.

August 11, 2017

A Pets Prayer:

If it should be, that I grow frail and weak,
And pain should keep me from my sleep,
Then, you must do what must be done
For this, the last battle, can't be won.
Don't let your grief stay your hand,
For this day more than the rest,
Your love and friendship stand the test.
We've had so many years,
What is to come can hold no fear.
You'd not want me to suffer, so
When the time comes, please let me go.
Take me where my needs they'll tend,
Only, stay with me to the end
And hold me firm and speak to me
Until my eyes no longer see.
I know in time you'll see it is a kindness you do for me
Although my tail its last has waved,
From pain and suffering I've been saved.
Don't grieve it should be you who this thing decides to do.
We've been so close, we two, these years,
Don't let your heart hold tears.
SMILE, FOR WE WALKED TOGETHER FOR AWHILE.

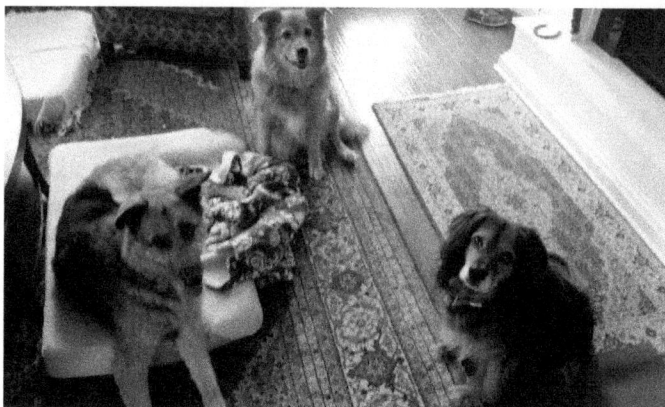

Sandy, Annie and Buddy

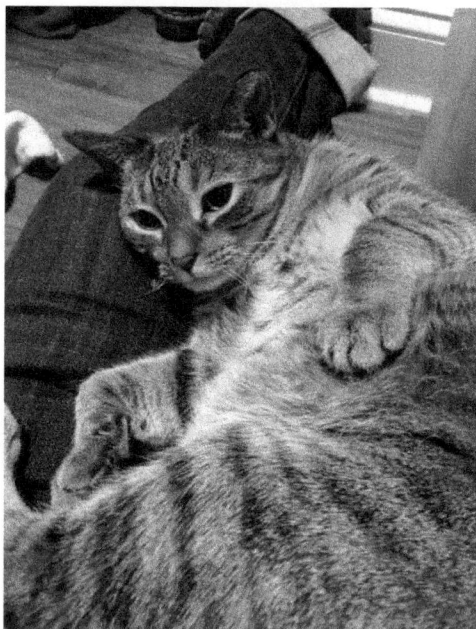

Tipper

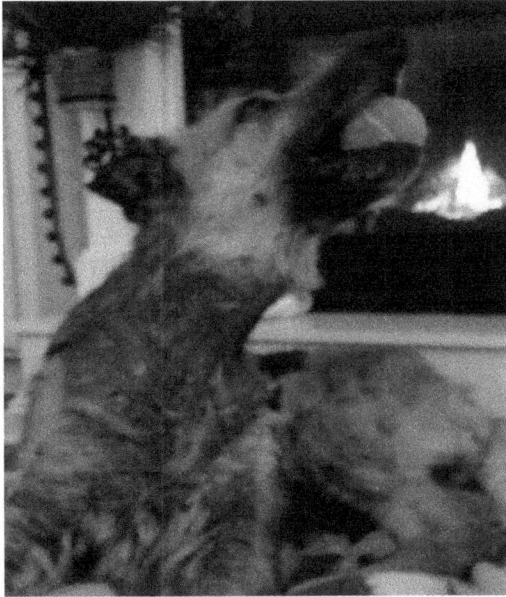

Sandy with her ball

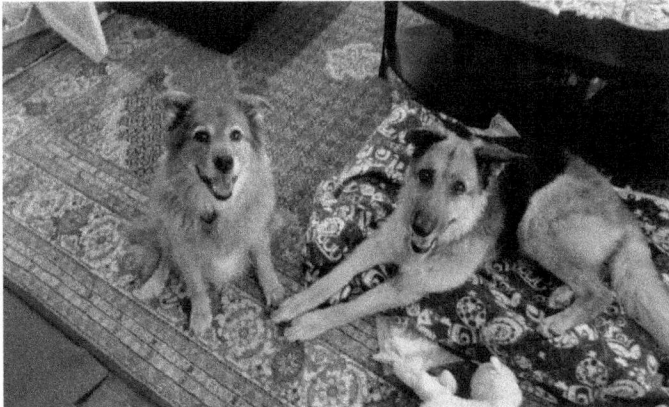

Annie and Sandy

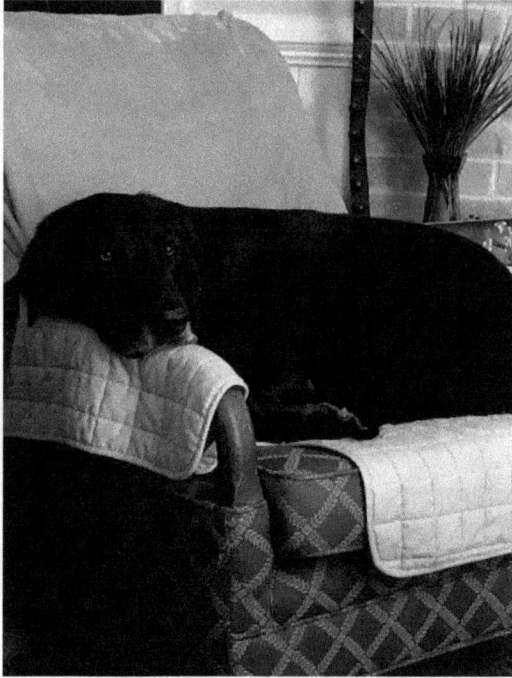

Cash in his favorite chair

August 11, 2017

Written by Carol Albrecht, a faithful and loving friend to Sandy and to Sandy's family.

Sandy,

Oh Lord, in your mercy, be and abide with Sandy and her family as they travel this week. We pray that the memories created here and now last the lifetime they have been given. Lord we are so very grateful for the love we have shared and the lessons we have learned in these brief months with Sandy. The child of your heart survived hardship and betrayal until finally brought to safety and life with her mom and dad. We are grateful for the time we have been given.

Sandy, I see you. I see you and the day is fresh, the sky full of promise, the grass soft and cool beneath your feet. I call your name. my voice floats on summer air!

"My dad" is close. The warmth of his presence as familiar and welcome as the sun against the earth. He knows my weight, the fraility of my body with the same understanding that I know and trust the strength of his arms. Our hearts an echo. My head against his chest, his calm sinks into my bones.

It is peaceful here. I watch the shadows. My ears twitch at the scuff of mama's slippered feet. Joy! Mama kneels beside my "your bed". Her scent washes over me, oh the relief, gentle massage on tired muscles. Mama lifts and strokes my big soft paws. She knows each pad, each toe, what feels good, what is scary. Mama, "my mom", rests her hand upon my head, caressing my ears. She leans close, inhaling the soft clean scent of my ruff. I close my eyes.

I feel in a dream the press of Annie's muzzle in my side and Buddy's whine, the caress of Tipper and Lulu's pink tongues against my eyelids.

And I am home.

Oh Lord, in your mercy, hear my prayer.

Sandy. Hear my voice! I call your name.

Accept this gift. I lift you up cradled in beautiful light; its pattern spun by grace. It is a gift, yours through time; the warp and weft of memory and love, hope and experience, woven through the months, days, and hours that your heart united with Mom's and Dad's.

Love's pink embrace casts the shadows from your eyes and forever binds your hearts. Amber's warm glow soothes aching muscles, tired bones. Heaven's blue to ease your pain, calms your fears.

Evening's lavender for quiet peace, gentle rest.
And the beautiful softest guiding white to light your path home.

Sandy,

I hear His voice calling on the breeze. You know him well, for you have heard the pitch and echo, felt the warmth of His love through Mom and Dad. His gift to you, to them. Time however brief, to know safety and compassion. And time to embrace life and the depth of Mom and Dad's love. Sandy, Our Lord, the Master of all creation calls. He calls you home. I lift you up.

Lord in your mercy, hear our prayer. Be with us as we release Sandy into your keeping.

Send your guardian angels to guide her safely across the bridge; that she might run on legs made strong again; that she may fly across the meadows and know the comfort of your heart, the warmth of your embrace.

And by your mercy and grace, comfort all those who mourn and are missing her this night.

I lift you up♪

~ Carol Albrecht

August 12, 2017

From Sandy's mom: I promise I will begin posting again when my heart isn't hurting so deeply and when I can do it in joy and not tears.

Love to all
Diana

August 14, 2017

To all of Sandy's Facebook Family,

Your thoughts and prayers for us are felt deeply. We are so thankful for your surrounding love and how much it helps us to be determined to get strong and carry on Sandy's message of hope. Our rooms feel empty and we listen for her panting and breathing that is in our heads and hearts.

Gabby is coming along and will have surgery on the 21st. She is a strange mix of Boz and Sandy. There will never be another Sandy, but we will spread her story and the story of all of you and how you loved her so much.

Thank you for taking this journey with us,

Mom and Dad.

August 18, 2017

One week. A week of being. Being broken, being sad, being empty, being guilty, being .... a week of knowing ...... knowing how deeply we loved her, knowing how much our other babies loved her, knowing Dr. Ruth loved her, knowing all of you loved her so very much. A week of hoping......hoping her life is full and healthy and blessed, hoping all of you know how much you meant to her and how much you mean to us. A week of being thankful for the gift of Sandy....thankful we got to be her mom and dad......thankful she put things in perspective, thankful she is back with her Creator.

August 20, 2017

Sandy, on her last morning, surrounded by all her toys, fast asleep.

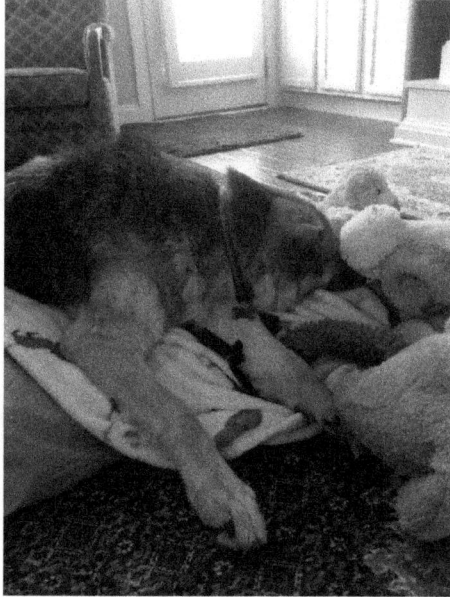

August 22, 2017

Mom's sweet cousin........ knows her heart! And to Lisa Hester Hall, this will stay with us forever.

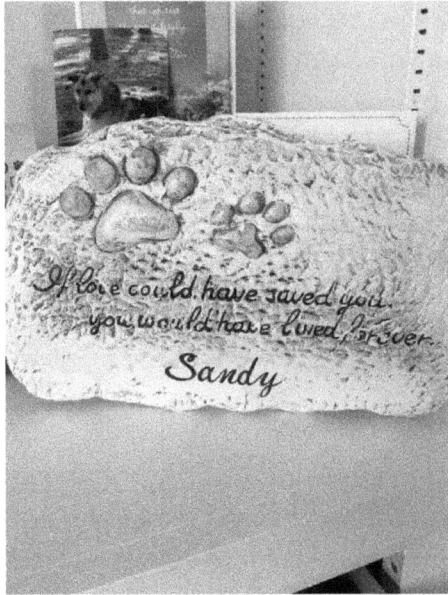

August 23, 2017

My heart was lifted today because I got to meet Gabby. She is 100% sweet and had some surgery yesterday. They removed a large mammary tumor and 3 smaller ones and spayed her yesterday so she's feeling pretty rough. It was healing and heartbreaking at the same time to feel her fur and rub her head. She is in a super wonderful home where she will be so loved and so well cared for. Her predecessors were Boz and Maggie and Pearl, all German Shepherds who took pieces of Sandy's aunt and uncle with them over the rainbow. She was rescued by them from a situation of serious neglect.

She is a source of healing for me and I hope she will be for all of you. Missing Sandy has been all consuming, the tears are not constant now, the ache not quite so acute ...... it's the emptiness and just plain old grief. Blessed to be able to be with family and Gabby.
I cannot thank each of you although I wish I could. I want you to know we read your comments. We read as much as we can before the tears

cloud our eyes and we resume when we feel stronger. Thank you seems inadequate. Sandy and all of you have changed our lives. When the world is so torn and the hatred so fierce we are blessed with the ability to love our animals and participate with you in sharing our love. For this we are grateful and blessed.

August 28, 2017

Hello all of you wonderful, faithful Sandy friends. Here is an update on Gabby:

The tumors that were removed were malignant, but they were all stage 1 level 1 and the vet believes they got it all. She will have to be monitored for these mammary tumors the rest of her life.
Gabby apparently lived quite a while on her own or under a house or deck. She has tried several times to claw her way through shrubbery to get under my sister's deck. She has some fear aggression and for no apparent reason will snap or put her mouth on your hand...

She has not really bitten, and does not show this behavior to my sister or her husband but does with me and my niece and nephew (who are adults and dog lovers). As a result she will go to a professional dog behaviorist after the sutures from her surgery are removed. She will go through training and so will the rest of the family to learn how to help her overcome this behavior. Her stress levels have been high with all the drastic changes in her life over the past three or four weeks so it is possible she is fearful of many things at this point. She is in the best home any dog could ever want and we will all love her through this process.

On another subject, Mom and Dad are working hard to adjust to life without Sandy. Mom has even volunteered to help in Texas through the efforts of Best Friends. We pray all of your pets who have evolved into loving beings in the next journey will watch over the animals who are drowning, who are alone, who are hungry and who are afraid.

August 30, 2017

Just want to let all of you know that I am on call for being notified by Best Friends to help in Texas. Will keep you posted if there are developments. In the meantime, Best Friends has set up a special fund for Harvey animals so visit www.bestfriends.org if you want more info. I refer to them because I know their work and trust them implicitly to make good judgment and use funding as intended.

Praying for all the horses and cattle and pets and the lost and scared animals. So very thankful for the human kindness being shown by people in Texas from all over our nation. Hoping Sandy may have inspired someone to save an animal.

So thankful our dogs and grand dogs and cats and horse are safe.

September 3, 2017

Friends. I need your help. The Houston SPCA has refused to let Best Friends take in the animals they have and the SPCA is a kill shelter. I need every one of Sandy's friends to sign this petition as many dogs are in danger of being euthanized.

Help save the pets in Hurricane Harvey!

People are risking their lives to rescue Harvey pets, yet some may go to shelters where they may be killed.

Please sign the below petition in our blog post to hold the Houston SPCA accountable for these lifesaving guarantees for animals rescued from Hurricane Harvey.

Yesterday the Best Friends Animal Society team on the ground in Texas arrived in Beaumont. Beaumont is one of the of the hardest hit areas by Hurricane Harvey and is struggling to provide basic services – the entire community lost access to clean water. The animals rescued from the area were being housed at a pavilion-type shelter set up at the Ford Center. The reports from our team on the ground late yesterday were that the animals were in dire need of basic medical care, and the heat was taking its toll.

The Houston SPCA obtained the memorandum of understanding (MOU) from local officials to serve as the small animal lead at the Ford Center. That's when the rumors began to swirl.

The Houston SPCA has a history of a lack of transparency around consistent reporting regarding the outcomes of the animals entering their care. They have questionable policies regarding pit bull type dogs and have received continued criticism from the animal welfare around these policies. So it's understandable that the rescue community and other pet-loving members of the public, aware of the Houston SPCA's history, would be worried about what was taking place with the pets in Beaumont.

We contacted the Houston SPCA and spoke with the organization's President, Patti Mercer. Knowing the Houston SPCA is already stretched thin from their necessary work in Houston, Best Friends offered to relieve them of the responsibility in Beaumont and take over the MOU to provide care and reunion efforts for the animals rescued in Beaumont. This offer was denied.

We then offered assistance and general help for the animals of Beaumont to the Houston SPCA, but this offer for help was also declined. While Ms. Mercer did verbally commit to at least a 30 day hold for the animals of Beaumont to be reunited with their owners, our attempts to determine if there would be an adoption guarantee for

these animals regardless of where they might be transferred failed –
we were told by Ms. Mercer to wait for a "press release" and she was
unwilling to put anything in writing to us. The list of possible receiving
agencies for these animals that she cited are not known for their
commitment to no-kill policies.

We detailed the expectations Best Friends has set for ourselves for
animals we rescue from this storm, and asked the Houston SPCA to
commit to the same, in writing.

Minimum 30-day stray hold so owners can reunite with their pets.
Proactive pursuit of families and reunion of all pets displaced by
Harvey.
A clear, transparent operation that offers an appropriate standard of
care.
A guarantee for a positive outcome for all animals rescued. In other
words, that all the animals in Beaumont are either reunited with their
families; adopted into a loving home; or are transferred to an agency
that will guarantee a no-kill outcome.
Sharing of raw data so that the above points can be audited and
confirmed by interested parties.

Ms. Mercer refused to put these simple commitments and
procedures in writing, and again she referred us to a yet-to-be-made
press release. We advised her that her personal word in writing to us
would do more to allay the public's concerns than a press release, but
again Ms. Mercer declined. Without this in writing, Best Friends does
not feel comfortable with what is happening in Beaumont, or
anywhere else the Houston SPCA is rescuing pets.

Whether it is a time of disaster or not, organizations that rescue
animals need to be held accountable by the communities they serve.
Best Friends is committed to helping the animals of Texas and will not
back down.

Please click here to sign a petition to hold Houston SPCA to these simple life-saving guarantees.

Help save the pets in Hurricane Harvey. People are risking their lives to rescue Harvey pets, yet some may go to shelters where they may be killed.

HOUSTON, HURRICANE HARVEY, TEXAS

https://www.change.org/p/patti-mercer-president-of-the-houston-spca-demand-houston-spca

September 4, 2017

I got the email today from Best Friends to sign up for volunteering in Houston. Will make a decision at the end of this week when I can go and will be there for 5 to 7 days. Have to figure out air travel, car rental and lodging. They are caring for over 500 animals, so their volunteers are coming in to help. Would love your energies and prayers for making this journey. More to come at the end of the week.

For Janice, the most gracious soul who has offered to assist me in my travel to Houston, I will send my info.

And to Sandy's friends in Texas, I welcome input about where and where not to stay near Conroe.

This will be a journey of faith!

September 6, 2017

To all of Sandy's Facebook Family. Mom, Diana/me will wait until after the path of this next hurricane is better defined before she makes air travel plans. She has to be in Richmond, Va. for a wedding on Sept 30th.

If any of you are interested or desire to go and have 5 or six days to spare, Mom would love the company. There are many, many jobs to be done, and it was looking even more urgent to help according to the job schedule of the intake center in Texas. Mom is going to try to negotiate a stay at one of the nearby hotels using her AAA membership. Flexibility with departure and arrival, and returning are making the trip less expensive, with air tickets around $360 round trip, we hope.

Many thanks to Sandy's friends in Texas for the heads-up about locations...... if you would pm me your contact info, it would surely be nice to have someone to call if I need something.
I promise to keep everyone updated as things get planned
Looks like there are a couple of hurricanes lurking and we pray hard that they don't gain strength and cause such destruction and loss of life.

September 6, 2017

Missing Sandy a lot today. Gabby is doing well with healing. She's a sweet girl who somehow ended up alone and afraid. She has some fear issues to overcome, but she is in the most loving and supportive home one could ask for.

We try hard not to think about that last day, but at times during each day, we miss the feel of her fur, the preparation of her meals, her loving kisses. And the tears come again.

September 7, 2017

If you are in any proximity to Atlanta or Jacksonville, I need your help. I'm working with Best Friends to find volunteers to drive animals to safety. They are ready to be picked up in Jacksonville. If you can help, please text me at 8045132083 so I can send the information to you for contacting Best Friends immediately. Please share.

<u>September 8, 2017</u>

Due to the intense need for help evacuating animals from Florida, I will be driving a cargo van to Atlanta on Sunday to pick up animals and transport them to Virginia. Best Friends called today and need this now versus going to Texas. I still may need to go to Texas or Florida after the storm, but we will hit the road Saturday pm to get to Atlanta for a pick-up and drive back to VA. Please know that Best Friends is accepting volunteers even if you've never volunteered before. Go to www.bestfriends.org, and it will walk you through how to sign up.

Thank you all for your encouragement and prayers. It is a bittersweet revelation at age 64 that animal rescue was what I should have started in my 20s. Better late than never.
Stay safe, and know how much Michael and I honor what you did for Sandy and are doing for all these animals in terrible danger.

Sandy continues her influence. Mom and Dad leave tomorrow a.m. to travel to Atlanta, GA, in a cargo van to pick up animals in Atlanta that have been transported out of Florida. They will then travel to Virginia to deliver these babies to safe havens.
It dawned on me that some people may not understand rescue and so don't volunteer. Here are things that have to be done in a rescue mission:

After the animals are rescued, put into shelter and receive veterinary care, they need to be fed. Food needs to be taken to the feeding set-up. Food needs to be received from donations and put into storage. Food needs to be inventoried and entered into the data system. Animals with identification need to be cataloged and entered into the data system. Animals with no ID and no chip must be given identification numbers and descriptions and entered into the data system. Someone must put tags on. Someone must walk each dog. Someone delivers food bowls. Someone picks up food bowls. Someone fills water bowls, and someone gives meds.

These "someones" are the volunteers. Many answer phones, and many follow up and help coordinate the arrivals and departures of animals. Many have to help manage his process. You don't have to be a previous volunteer to become one now. All hands on deck is the byword of the day and the days to come.

We leave tomorrow with a van to drive to Atlanta to pick up a vanload of animals to take to Virginia. There are different legs of each journey, and many volunteers are needed to drive one leg to another. If you are able to help with any of these small tasks that make this job so very important, please sign up at <u>bestfriends.org</u> to help. You are needed.

It's 2:29 am on 9/11/17. Thanks to all of Sandy's wonderful Facebook Family, Mom and Dad, with the help of Sandy's auntie, were able to transport 8 sweet dogs from Atlanta to Fairfax, VA, in conjunction with helping to clear Best Friends shelter to make way for Hurricane Irma's victims. It was a long two days but worth every moment. Eight fur babies are now in a wonderful shelter awaiting adoption in Fairfax, Va., and eight spots are open for saving eight more!

Sandy's Legacy

September 15, 2017

Dear friends of Sandy,

Mom and Dad went out to dinner tonight and ran into Lexi, our wonderful vet tech who was with us through thick and thin and kind enough to come hold Mom at the hardest time. It made us think of what a loving and kind dog Sandy was and how lucky we were to rescue such a wonderful animal. She was magnificent in her crippled body, but the most beautiful thing was her heart and the wonderful things she taught us. For a year and a half, she was the number one priority in our household. That lesson was life-changing. The oriental silk and wool rug where she slept became so unimportant. The early rising to her panting to go outside became a healthy practice. The patience it took to get her to eat and to help her outside was something we needed to learn to slow down and smell the flowers and watch the birds and butterflies. She showed us the supreme forgiveness because she had every reason to despise humans for all she had endured. But, she loved us. She was a gentle, sweet, loving, wonderful part of our lives, and she touched so many. What a blessing and what a champion!

September 18, 2017

We were just today able to sort through Sandy's things that we put away in the garage. Her bedding still smelled like her and we just put it in the washer.

So, we would like to know if any of her Facebook family needs wheels for a 96-pound dog. We were blessed to be able to get them with her GoFundMe page and want to pass them on to a beloved dog who needs them. Please private message me with information if you need them.

Thank you.

September 22, 2017

Sandy's family. Today was a day of disappointment for us. We are deeply ashamed that Virginia Tech would choose to honor a man who chose to abuse dogs to such degrees that are indescribable. Mom and Dad are both Virginians by birth and lived there a long time. Mom also had the opportunity to care for some of the Vick(tory)dogs when volunteering at Best Friends. We are dismayed that a state college would choose to honor a person of his character, and yet we are grateful that his despicable behavior has led to greater knowledge of abused dogs and animals. We choose to express our disgust by never watching another athletic event in which Virginia Tech participates.

September 27, 2017

The house is quiet, and we are missing Sandy. We miss seeing the peace in her eyes when lying on the rug in the den. We miss her whining when she wanted us to take her out. We miss the cold black nose that rubbed our hands. We miss her presence, and we are grateful for having the privilege of being her people, even if it was for just a while. We hope everyone in her Facebook family will stay in touch with us.

October 3, 2017

We thought you'd like to know about Gabby and her progress. For those of you who don't know who Gabby is, it goes like this: Mom saw a post by a friend on Facebook about a female German Shepherd who had crawled up their driveway weak and covered in ticks and fleas and who had been sprayed by a skunk. Mom's friends kept her and bathed and cleaned her for a week in spite of having three large dogs and several horses. They knew they couldn't take care of her, too, so they posted her on Facebook and took her to the Powhatan Virginia Animal Control. No one claimed her. Mom told her sister, who was Bozzie's and Maggie's and Pearl's mom, about this dog. Bozzie and Pearl had both crossed the Rainbow Bridge in the past 6 months, and Maggie had crossed a year before.

So Mom's sister and brother-in-law went to see this homeless dog, and their hearts melted. She had ehrlichiosis and was 30 some pounds underweight. But she found a wonderful new mom and dad and couldn't ask for a better home, complete with a huge fenced yard and anything she needs. She had never been socialized, and so Mom's sister and her husband hired a highly trained and certified dog trainer who has worked miracles in 6 weeks. Gabby has some fear aggression and is gradually increasing her circle of people that she trusts. She is extremely smart and so sweet. Her shoulders are genetically bad but she gets the meds she needs and has gained 15 pounds! She did extremely well with Mom and Dad visiting this past weekend and loves to have a job! So Sandy's legacy lives on in Gabby and in each of the animals' lives that have been rescued or cared for by her Facebook Family.

Mom and Dad's lives have changed drastically without Sandy, and they find themselves at loose ends some days. Buddy and Annie are getting extra love and attention, and Annie will go to have her teeth cleaned next week. Tipper and Lulu are such creatures of habit and love their dogs! We think of all of you so many times during any given day and, in particular, these past two days. We count our blessings to have been touched by each of you and know you all join us in beseeching God and the universe to strengthen our resolve to be more loving and kind, especially in the aftermath of our national tragedy. None of us is promised tomorrow, and so it is important to send our love to all of you.

Here is Gabby enjoying the fresh air.

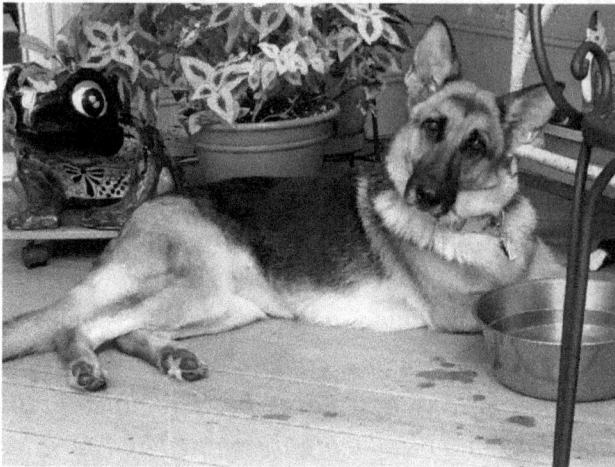

October 10, 2017

Hello Sandy's Facebook Family. Each one of us that has ever suffered the loss of a beloved pet or human family loved one knows how this goes. Your days begin to fill with tasks and being busy and sometimes just doing things to keep you busy, and then, WHAM, your heart wrenches, and you have an empty spot that nothing will fill. Well, today was like that. Annie was at the vet having her teeth cleaned, and Buddy retreated to his bed. The den felt so empty. The big bed where Sandy stayed most of the time is cleaned and put away, and then the guilt starts to creep in. The questions of, "Did we do the right thing?", "Was she ready?", "Would she still be lying here peacefully?", "Did we read her face wrong?" The tortuous guilt is creeping in on all we believed and trying to tear at our hearts.

Then, totally unexpectedly, a box arrives in the mail. A gift in memory of Sandy from someone very special to Mom and Dad. And the answer to all the imposition of guilt is clearly yes, we did what we promised her and guided her to a place where she is free, just like all of us will be one day. Oh, that we could each be blessed with the end of life in peace and understanding. Until then, we are charged with dominion over the living things that cannot speak for themselves. We will send each other strength and love, and total understanding because these wonderful pets have made us better people. Blessings to all of you. We miss every single comment and want you to know that the book will begin this week. Pray for the people and animals in harm's way and pay it forward. Sandy would want that.

October 25, 2017

Facebook Family,

Although we have had a couple of people who needed carts for their dogs, as yet, we have not been able to donate them to a needy dog due to the measurements of the wheels.

Sandy's cart was made by Eddie's wheels and custom fit for her. If you need wheels and think your dog might fit, please go to Eddie's Wheels website and measure your dog according to the instructions. If you believe hers might work, please compare it to her measurements below and let us know.

Here are the details on Sandy's cart. Keep in mind, if the new dog's measurements are bigger than measurements C or any of the E's, then the cart won't fit. The width of the cart and the size of the saddle loop are not adjustable. It is a variable axle cart with stirrups.

A: 26 1/2
B: 16
C: 8
D: 17
E shoulders: 8 3/4

E ribs: 8 1/4
E rump: 8 ¼

November 4, 2017

It's November and hard to believe it! An update on Gabby. She has gained 15 pounds since rescue and is one happy and loved girl. She is still working with a trainer on her fear aggression but seldom exhibits it and never to her new mom or dad, just new people. She has the typical fear aggression with some people: when they turn to walk away she will do her herding nip. However if she's given a job, to sit or stay she doesn't do it. It's obvious she lived on her own for quite a while. She's very loved and Mom loves spending time with her!

We miss hearing from all of you and we miss that wonderful head tossing stubborn beautiful girl Sandy! She lives every day in our hearts and makes us remember the glass half full not half empty!
We send our love and thanks to all of you and want you to know how much you all filled our hearts throughout Sandy's journey.

November 11, 2017

Mom has to share this. Sandy's bed was washed and put away in the garage. Long story short.... mom and dad put Buddy's and Annie's beds in garage while cleaning rugs and when dad brought them back in he brought Sandy's instead of Buddy's. There was a large amount of sniffing done by everyone including Tipper, and mom decided Sandy would like it if Buddy had her bed. So he's all curled up and fast asleep. Mom and dad have submitted applications to volunteer at Saving Grace Animal Rescue so we will keep you posted.

November 14, 2017

Hello FB family. We learned that there is an adopted GSD named Queenie who can possibly measure to fit Sandy's wheels. We read about her in The Dodo FB Page. We would love to have help getting in touch with her new mom to see if she could measure Queenie and we could ship our Eddie's Wheels to her. If you know how we can contact her, please let us know.

Happy Thanksgiving and blessings to all. We will post again soon.

Mom

November 19, 2017

We have now found out that Queenie has already received wheels from a generous donor. So, please share and let us know if a dog in need can use Sandy's wheels.

Still need help finding Queenie to see if she needs / can use Sandy's wheels. Any and all help is greatly appreciated! Also wanted to let all of you know that Dr. Ruth West, our Dr. Ruth, came by to see us the other day and we have missed her so much. Annie and Buddy were very happy to see her and she brought them special treats! She is a blessing on this earth!

Sending our prayers for your safe travels and bountiful goodness on this Thanksgiving.

December 3, 2017

Season's greetings to all of you! We have been busy singing and doing the Christmas things but haven't forgotten about our big plan for 2018 which is to finish and publish Sandy's book. In the meantime, Mom and Dad will be downsizing a bit but will keep all of you posted. Buddy has been diagnosed with a heart condition and suspicious spots on his lungs so he is on heart meds and we are keeping a close eye on him. He's eating well and very happy so things don't look too grim right now. Thought we share this lovely photo of Sandy from last Christmas.

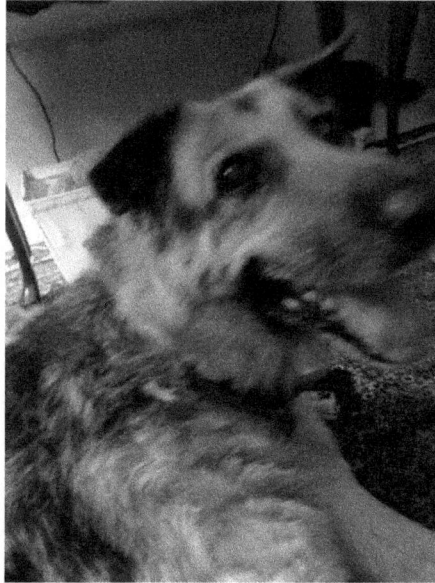

December 16, 2017

Mom and Dad and Annie and Buddy and Tipper and Lulu send their wishes for the merriest and most blessed Christmas. Donations were made this Christmas in memory of Sandy to several places. With each donation we remembered all of you who made her last year and a half of life so incredibly good. God is doG spelled backwards. Love to each one of you, your families and your fur babies.

December 31, 2017

Happy New Year form Sandy's mom and dad! May you always know how much you are loved and appreciated. May you always be as forgiving as Sandy was, may you be strong and courageous like she was and may 2018 carry you forward with warm sweet memories.

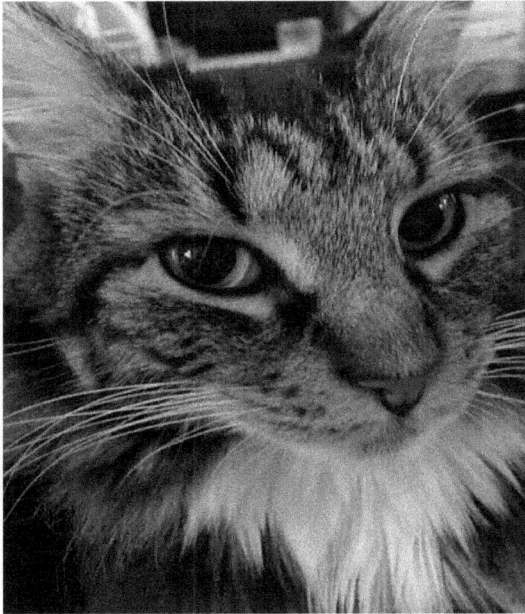

Lulu

January 10, 2018

Happy New Year to all her family and many blessings on you. Here's to a year of more rescues and working to make the lives of animals better. Hug your fur babies tonight... lots to tell all of you when we settle in to 2018!

January 14, 2018

Christmas was a bit nostalgic without our beautiful girl. To top it off, Mom blew out her right knee on Christmas Eve. It was a mad rush to get X-rays and MRI before year end. Cortisone shots will carry mom through for the next few months then it will have to be taken care of. Another major change in mom's and dad's lives is downsizing; PM mom if you want to know details.

The east has been hit hard with bitter cold again so we think of all the animals who are lost or alone and pray they will find shelter and be kept from the bitter cold. Stay warm.

January 14, 2018

OK, Sandy's family. It's time to get to work. I received this post from one of Sandy's followers and am trusting that Sandy's Facebook family can help. I have the name of the person who posted this and am in touch with her.
Please, please let's help with this!

From Sandy's friend,

Does anyone have any contacts with a German shepherd rescue specializing in older sheps? A plus if they have experience with DM. I have an older shepherd, maybe 8ish that came in as a stray that was possibly hit by car. He was found on the side of the road not able to use his rear end.

We did full X-rays. No broken bones. No scrapes to suggest a hit by car. It has been decided that he most likely has DM. He has a microchip but the owners have failed to respond to calls, messages, or certified mail. I am really hoping that they did not get tired of him and just dump him. He is facing euthanasia if I cannot find a rescue group to take him. The local rescue group who originally brought him in will not be able to take care of his needs.

He is a sweet dog to me; however, he has growled when we have tried to do things he doesn't like. Unsure if it is because of pain or just because he has not been socialized well. The first day he was sad and wanted to be left alone. After feeding him and giving him steroids, he has perked up! He is able to stand-ish and wags his tail in greeting when I go to take him out. I have to use a sling to steady him. The right leg has some control, but he can't do much with the left. He let me pick him up and maneuver him into a cart to help him walk. However, it was too short, so we had to go back to the sling. He is able to swing his back legs and get going but needs help staying steady.

I would love to save this guy who was found broken on the side of the road. I do not want to give up on him, even with his flaws. So please if anyone has contacts please tag them in this post! A lot of specifics cannot be named due to legality reasons, but I will do my best to answer them. He is located in Cincinnati, Ohio.

January 25, 2018

Hello all. Praying all of you are avoiding the flu and the upper respiratory crud that invaded our household the past two weeks. Strangest "cold" mom's ever had! All in her head and sinuses. Thankful for tissues with lotion. Annie and Buddy are doing fine. Bud is slowing down a bit but still excited when treats are offered or some other dog comes by. Gabby has rounded the corner and become very happy and comfortable in her home. She is very affectionate and a German Shepherd dog in every sense of the word. Some of her "airs" and mannerisms are big reminders of Sandy. For Christmas, Rachael, Sandy's human sister, gave mom an incredible book of pictures she came and took and took pieces of Sandy's posts to go with them. It is on the coffee table and mom will be posting some for all to see. The book mom is writing is getting done, slowly but getting there. Lots to edit (grammar and misspelling) due to mom's words just flowing out of her head too fast and not doing spell check before posting.

We follow Trio Animal Foundation in Facebook and stay amazed at the miracles they manage. We follow several others too and are so thankful for social media because it is saving the lives of animals every day. So remember to share the Facebook posts you see where organizations are working so hard to Save Them All ...... the goal of Best Friends Animal Sanctuary is to have no more homeless pets by 2022. We must stay strong and with Sandy's spirit urging us on, WE CAN DO THIS!"

February 16, 2018

As I sit here tonight paging through the photographs Sandy's human sister took, it made me think that about Sandy's lessons of hope. The past week has been full of despair and gut wrenching loss of innocents and innocence. What will we all choose to take from this? Will we point fingers and waste words while someone else plots to take more hope from us? What will we choose to think? Will we blame mental health issues while someone else posts threats to which we pay no attention? What will we choose to do? Will we pray for wisdom and wait?

The wisdom of an abused and neglected soul whose rescue inspired hope and joy and awareness tells me that the action of rescue is needed by all of us. We all need to rescue hope, to stand for the voiceless and the innocent. Who will stand for them and who will choose the commitment it will take to stop school violence? What will we choose to say? Will we speak with rational loving voices who value the most precious gift of life........ or will we scroll down the pages of the lives lost and think there is nothing we can do? Hope says we won't. Hope says we will lift up our voices to plead for those who represent us to rid us of the plague of automatic weapons? Hope says our selfish needs to be powerful will be balanced by our understanding of the power of love and of life.

March 13, 2018

This is a long overdue update / greeting; so much has been going on and mom has been remiss in keeping all informed. Dad and mom have re-settled in Virginia and the move has occupied us for a long time. All is finally settled in and Buddy, Annie, Tipper and Lulu are doing fine. Buddy's heart murmur is slowing him down and his heart is enlarged but he's still a very happy boy! We are in an apartment until we find the right house.

Gabby, who would have been Sandy's cousin, has come such a long way and is just so sweet around children and finally not feeling like she has to be so guarded.

Sandy's St. Francis and her memorial stone are right here with mom and dad, and the beautiful photo book that Sandy's human sister gave mom and dad for Christmas is right on the coffee table. There is not a day that goes by that we don't think of her and miss her.

Mom misses being in touch with all of you, so she will be updating more often and setting chapter goals for Sandy's story.

Love to each one of you. You are not forgotten!

March 14, 2018

87! 87 pages done in the draft of Sandy's book! Nowhere near finished, but the die is cast and the work continues. It is bittersweet to read posts from 2016, but oh, what joy she brought to us.

Who knew that a bedraggled mange-covered creature could form such a family as all of you! So very blessed.

April 2, 2018

Hate to ask, but please ask St Francis and St. Anthony and all the powers of the universe to bring Lulu home. She slipped out last Tuesday when we were carrying groceries in. Annie, Buddy and Tipper miss her, and mom has been about crazed looking for her. She is chipped, and we've reported her as missing. We have done the following:

Posted on numerous social media including Nextdoor and Paw Boost
Set our clothes and shoes outside.
Set her blanket outside.
Called the local vet office.
Put posters up.
Called the county animal "shelter."
Knocked on doors.
Ridden through adjoining neighborhoods and put up signs, and gave out our info.
Called her every two to three hours.
Set a trap with her treats and mackerel.
Monitor trap every daybreak, noon and evening and late night.
Set out her litter box.
Consulted with cat rescuers.
Made people who feed feral cats around here aware.
Have been under every bush and tree in the complex.
We do have a very territorial outdoor kitty who lives next door to us.
Prayed and prayed and have been trying so hard not to give up.

April 2, 2018

Sandy's forever family. Sandy and all of your prayers worked within an hour! Lulu has been gone for a week. She was seen going into the storm drain by neighbors. I took her treat bag, shook it, and called into the drain softly, and she is home. A miracle and an answer to so many wonderful prayers. I'll never be able to thank you.

April 24, 2018

Hello all. We are thankful to have finally made a decision about where we will live and have been consumed with the downsizing thing. Of course, we have continued to be thankful for finding Lulu, and she is back to normal, minus a pound or two. As many of you know, Annie and Buddy are seniors, so they have slowed down considerably. Buddy has a very enlarged heart, and for some reason, one lung has collapsed. He is still eating and on 3 meds for his heart. He still wags and goes about life very slowly. We know the time is near when he will not be having a good time anymore, and as you all know so well, mom and dad will be broken again for a while. Mom stays tuned in to numerous rescues and Sandy's book is coming, she promises.

Most of all, we miss being in touch with each one of you. Your kindness and support will never be forgotten. As the book comes along, mom will be asking for permission from each of you to use your name in the printed copy. Mom will send a post when it's time so a log can be kept of each of your names. An orderly apartment doesn't allow for much space to organize pictures and stuff for the book, so soon, we will be able to spread out.

Love and blessings to all of you!

May 4, 2018

Sandy's brother Buddy is failing quickly. It's so hard because we don't want him to struggle and we are trusting he will let us know when he's ready to go be with Sandy. All prayers and energies of love are appreciated. I want to be strong but my heart hurts.

May 6, 2018

Sandy's family; Buddy's heart is very enlarged, and his breathing is shallow. He sleeps most of the time. Our vet, at Sycamore Veterinary Hospital, has been wonderful and we are taking it a day at a time, knowing he is at risk for a heart attack, and watching him closely. Mom and Dad thank each of you for all the love and support and prayers. We will be spending the next days letting him have anything he wants. Today was ham and chicken.

Mom and dad know that most of you have gone through losing a fur baby, if not several. Our vet is wise and says no matter how they leave us or when, we are ripped apart and there is no getting around it. Each pet leaves us with incredible grief but many blessings while they are here. In the Bible, it says that God gave man dominion over all the animals. Our prayer is to use this with wisdom and grace and courage.

May 9, 2018

Today our Buddy was released from shallow breath and a diseased heart. Mom and dad and Annie were with him. He was peaceful and relaxed with his head in Mom's hand. Breathe, sweet boy. Our tears are for ourselves and our trust is in the heavens where Sandy met you and we will be together again.

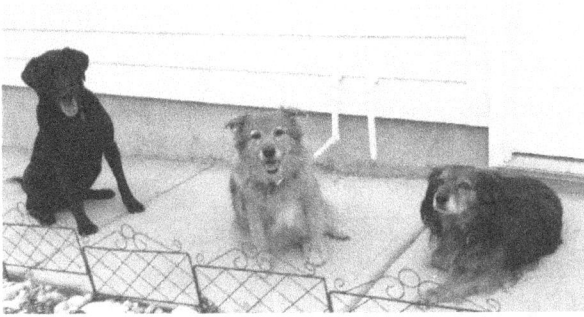

Cash, Annie and Buddy

May 16, 2018

Well. Mom and dad are still working at the new normal without Sandy and without Buddy. Our veterinarian had the wisest words for us in deciding to help Buddy on to the next journey. She said that it doesn't matter if you pick the date or the date picks you; it is a gut-wrenching, all enveloping and overwhelming feeling when you lose them. You cannot avoid it. The only thing you can do is walk through it. With your kind words and healing prayers, we are walking, sometimes more quickly than others. We want all of you to know that we are acutely aware of this path, so many of you have had to walk already, and some of you who are facing the gate to this path. Your sorrow and angst are ours, too, and we want to let you know Sandy's family is never very far from our thoughts. It is such a gift in this world of division that we have all come together to feel connected because of one sweet girl named Sandy. How blessed we are, and it helps us each day to remember to take joy into our being every time it is available.

May 30, 2018

Mom and Dad and Annie and Tipper and Lulu send our love to all of you. Sometimes life just gets in the way of all good intentions, but we are working on the book. M and D are the proud holders now of their

Medicare cards and we will have new digs by the end of June. Gabby is thriving and loves Mom, who is her "Auntie". Once we settle, we will look to find just the right rescue to work well in our household, where will hope to continue to spread the love. We miss our Buddy and our Sandy and will post pictures of them dogs once we unpack. Mom especially misses each of you but is excited about sharing photos of Sandy soon that have never been seen. Going through hundreds trying to find the right ones for the book.

Mom knows she is overdue for posting. It's a busy month of moving. However, we need your help. A friend of Mom's has rescued a pit mix and lives outside of Atlanta. The poor thing was traumatized by being in a shelter and has been labeled as having behavioral issues and we are trying to find a rescue that can help with this. Mom's friend can't keep the dog but doesn't want the poor baby to be sent to a shelter where it will be traumatized again. Do any of Sandy's family know of a place near Atlanta or even a nearby state who could help????

June 16, 2018

Mom promises to be back soon. Moving and re -furnishing for next four weeks. She and dad think of you often. In fact, for Father's Day, Dad got shadow boxes of me and Buddy with our paw prints and pictures and collars. Sending love to all the dads and step dads and granddads out there!

Mom knows she is overdue on posting.

July 18, 2018

Sandy's family, we are all ok, just getting moved into our new home. We will not forget any of you! Just give mom a couple of weeks to get settled, and we will begin posting more often.

July 19, 2018

One more week, and mom will be set up in her new music room/office. The move is just on her mind so much and we are all hopeful that we will have time soon to move forward.

Just a quick update: mom found the neighbor's cat who had been missing for a week! And, always the animal lover, she took issue with the apartment management who warned all residents about feeding the feral cat colony. Residents were threatened with eviction if they fed the cats, so mom suggested they contact several different rescues that do spay and release. She's checking with one tomorrow to make sure they are aware. Some dog owners complained that the cats were dangerous to their dogs...onward !!!!

August 13, 2018

Hello Sandy's family. Mom is reaching out to all of you and asking all of you to share this message. I am not in the habit of posting about any of the rescues on Sandy's page. Tonight I am making an exception because there is a puppy who needs any and all prayers you can muster up. Your love and healing energies kept Sandy in such a good place emotionally and physically, and I KNOW you are the ones who kept me going so many times!

I am attaching the Facebook posts by Trio Animal Foundation. This is one of the rescues that I support for so many reasons. However, tonight, there is a German Shepherd who needs all of us. Thank you for indulging my request for your prayers, and send your angels to help this poor baby.

August 30, 2018

Well, we are unpacked and beginning to hang pictures and make it home. Wanted all of you to see that Sandy has a prominent place in our den and I look at her every day. I never fail to think about what a wonderful soul she was and how much she taught me. My office is set up minus a couple of things, but I'm ready to start back on the book. Most of all I want you all to know that I miss you. As Sandy's mom I became attached to so many of you and love the fact that I recognize your names and know you think of her too. I had to pick up meds for Annie yesterday at the vet and was parking when an elderly golden retriever was being carried in on a stretcher. I ached for the owners, and I cried when I got back in the car. I am so thankful to be able to love animals the way I do and to trust that they, too, never end but just become part of the eternal energy in a space of peace. I am thankful for each of you that shared our journey. It was and is life changing.

September 10, 2018

To Sandy's family and our friends: we are well stocked with non-perishables and water in anticipation of power outages and torrential rain. Mom has been in touch with Best Friends to see if there is anything she can do to help get animals out of the coastal areas of North Carolina and Virginia, so we are waiting to see if we can help. We are, as usual, hoping everyone will see that their pets are safe and making plans for how to care for them during and after this hurricane. If any of Sandy's family needs help with their pets, please let mom know so this unbelievable group of loving people can band together to get your animals to safety. We will do all we can, even if it is just spreading the word!! This hurricane Florence is no joke, so take good precautions!!

September 13, 2018

Mom is sharing a post she wrote on her own Facebook Page.:
There are so many times I see posts for animals and I don't feel Sandy's Page should be used as a vehicle to post about other animals very often. However, I've been reading about this baby for two days and felt led to pass on what I posted this evening about Jude. I know all of you who love Sandy so much will "get it". This is about Jude who is in the care of Shenandoah Shepherd Rescue.

I know many of my Facebook friends don't want to read or see the posts about lost or injured or abused dogs. I understand. I don't want to see them either. About 8 years ago I traveled to Utah to Best Friends Animal Sanctuary. It was here that I discovered the story of the 1970's hippies who set out to save all the lost and abandoned and mistreated animals. Their story of starting in a trailer in the canyons is worth reading about. (Www.bestfriends.org) It was here in Kanab Utah that I had a life changing experience. Had I been a millennial or any other post baby boomer age, I may have been able to discover my purpose in the early part of my life and education. However, I was part of the rise of women enough to break the glass ceiling, or so we thought, by becoming a corporate suit. Since my visit to volunteer at the Sanctuary I have pursued rescue and support of rescue at every turn. I am proud to say that I am part of the effort to Save Them All by 2022, the mission of Best Friends and their partners.

So I will continue to post the creatures that need our help. If I reach one more person, and help save one more life, it is worth losing every Facebook friend who chooses to "unfollow" me. I am blessed that my husband supports me in this and that he also has such great love and compassion for creatures.

And so, I post this about Jude, a beautiful creature of God who lay on a sidewalk for days while people passed him by. I'll never understand people who do that, nor do I want to. But today, he was rescued and being given the best care possible to let him know that he is loved even if it is for a few hours of his desperate life. These rescue organizations don't ask for you to pick up these dogs or clean up after them, they simply need financial help. Jude doesn't have a voice, so to the Friends I have who will read this, I will be his voice and the voice for those I know of who are God's creatures and are in need. Please send prayers for Jude and trust with me that Jude will know love if only for a little while.

September 14, 2018

Jude has gone to a place of pure love and no pain. Humans failed him for so long and then the angels that rescued him allowed him to know love for 24 hours. Thank you family for you expressions of love to him and your outreach to others about him. Our prayer here at our house is that lessons were learned through his suffering and if we succeeded in making even one person think twice about leaving a neglected dog to die, then Jude's passing is not in vain.

Update: as many of you know, mom and dad moved back to Midlothian Virginia. We had some very scary tornadoes today in the aftermath of Hurricane Florence. We are fine and didn't suffer any damage. In addition, just a word about the dogs and cats being rescued in North Carolina. Many of them are being sheltered at the state fairgrounds in Raleigh and some of the rescue shelters have cleared their shelters in order to take in these hurricane and flood victims. As was feared, many dogs were found in locked kennels in the more rural areas where Florence is causing tremendous flooding. Some dogs had literally been swimming for hours to stay alive.
Although most of us dog lovers consider this a horrible crime and cruelty to animals, there is obviously a significant population that believes it's ok to let your animals starve or drown. It's mom's most

fervent hope that Sandy's family can be ambassadors and advocates for these creatures who have no voice. We can do this in so many ways. We can volunteer, we can vote, we can share on social media, we can tell the stories when we are with friends or on the bus or the train. Every word we share about the plight of animals who are neglected and homeless is a step in the right direction.

Saving Grace Animal Shelter in Raleigh and Second Chance Rescue in Raleigh are at the forefront of the effort in North Carolina to educate those who leave animals to die. Best Friends in Utah, Georgia, and New York has a goal of no more homeless pets by 2022. Let's stand together and each one of us commit to saying or doing something every day to help these creatures. We are a powerful lot when we band together so as Sandy's family we can make a difference no matter how large or small!

Mom and dad have signed up for helping to transport dogs to shelters...... it's so easy and if this is something you'd like to do just go to doobert.com and it walks you through volunteering.

Prayers are needed for the animals who are still standing in water and waiting for someone to help them.

September 24, 2018

Mom is pretty excited! She finished the prologue today and did it with her new keyboard that connects by Bluetooth to her IPad! Progress!!!!!!

I hope and pray my proofreaders are still willing to do it!

Prologue- check
Dedication - check
1st 6 months - check

Making progress! Even saved her pictures to a flash drive!

A new chapter in rescue for me. Next weekend I will participate in transporting three precious pups to a shelter north of here. If you ever think you want to do something to help animals in need, but you can't foster or adopt, check out volunteering for Doobert. It's such a valuable service and requires so little. Doobert.com !!

October 24, 2018

Greetings all....... Mom (me) has been out of commission with an iPad that crashed and would not recover. Good news is that it is being replaced by Apple!!!!!!!!!!! So writing anything has been limited since the iPhone causes some issues with mom's hands.

With all the bomb scares and mass murders last week, we have been pausing to take stock of our own lives and offering prayers for all those that were slain, their families and friends, and their synagogue. Mom has taken initiative on her own to report and block all political Facebook sites for several reasons. She never knows if the site is legitimate or jacked by foreigners, and she is tired of the name calling, the lies, the bullying, and the misuse of social media. Our family knows it is time to take a stand for decency, for kindness, for honesty, and for consideration. What has happened to our country that we are repeating our own history? History that doesn't need repeating and does not represent who we need to be, it is disconcerting and scary.

On the bright side of life, mom has become an official transporter with Doobert and with Best Friends. And... hold on to your hats... we have a new family member. Dad is over the moon! And of course mom is too! Annie has loved it and the kitties are getting used to the idea. Pictures to come soon. Please know that we want to share details but we will only share when all is cleared up in the legal system. Neglect is a terrible thing. We are back doing what we do!!!!

December 2, 2018

Many thanks to those of you who have messaged me encouraging me to update!! Believe it or not I still have no iPad but have been promised by Apple that it will be here by next week. Major snafu's in getting problem resolved but a super customer care guy named Nick! While the laptop is gone, I've gone through cards and notes from Sandy's FB family. It's hard to believe we've lost Sandy and Buddy in less than two years. Sandy's pictures hang in our family room and never a day passes that I don't miss her.

Last Christmas, Sandy's auntie gave us a German Shepherd ornament, and I hung it on the tree today and felt her near. Annie has been a lonely girl without Sandy and Buddy, and we are in the midst of running tests to see if the Rimadyl is making her liver count bad. Third blood test this coming week. Most of all, we want all of you to know we miss you! Mom (me) misses your messages and posts and the daily interaction we shared. I started driving transports recently and hope to do more soon. Doobert is the transport organization I recently joined, and I am also approved by Best Friends to transport. It's very rewarding and not hard. Here's a picture of part of our Christmas mantel. Mom made the sign out of her grandmother's sewing table top. The strange man is back beside the fireplace and has an all-knowing look as if he knows Sandy's sweet spirit is looking at him.

December 16, 2018

It's a very long Apple story but mom still doesn't have her IPad and instead of Apple fixing the old one it looks like they will be sending a new one because of multiple messes on their part. However, we want to send our love and very merriest wishes to all of you for a blessed season of joy and peace. The house is looking like Christmas and it was a challenge to figure out the places to decorate! We had 14" of snow last weekend and frigid temperatures so we had an early white Christmas. Mom got to talk with one of the canine officers of our county who recently had to let his retired German Shepherd cross over that wondrous rainbow bridge. Mom shared Sandy's story with him and was happy to talk about her.

Our new addition is named Seamus and once the path is clear to assure he will never be neglected again and he gets healthy we will be able to share more info. We trust that Sandy and Buddy are with your fur babies who have gone to their next journey. May your hearts be full of joy knowing they have been met with open arms of angels and the Goodness of what waits for all of us.

December 17, 2018

It's here!!!!! And just to make things more complicated, we have to order a new keyboard because the new old one doesn't fit. But, we have the iPad!!!!

Our Christmas wish is that every dog and cat have a home, no more homeless or neglected or abused or lost or stolen animals. We send each of you our wishes for your peace.

Make me an instrument of thy peace
Where there is hatred, let me sow love, where there is injury, pardon,
Where there is doubt, Faith
Where there is despair, hope
Where there is darkness, light
Where there is sadness, joy
O Divine Master, grant that I may not so much seek to be consoled as to console,
To be understood, as to understand
To be loved, as to love
For it is in giving that we receive

It is in pardoning that we are pardoned,
And it is in dying that we are born to eternal life.
Prayer of St Francis of Assisi

December 25 2018

The blessings of Christmas to all of you!
Diana, Michael, Annie, Lulu, Tipper, Seamus.

Sending our wishes to all of you for joy today and tomorrow and always. Merry Christmas Sandy's FB family!

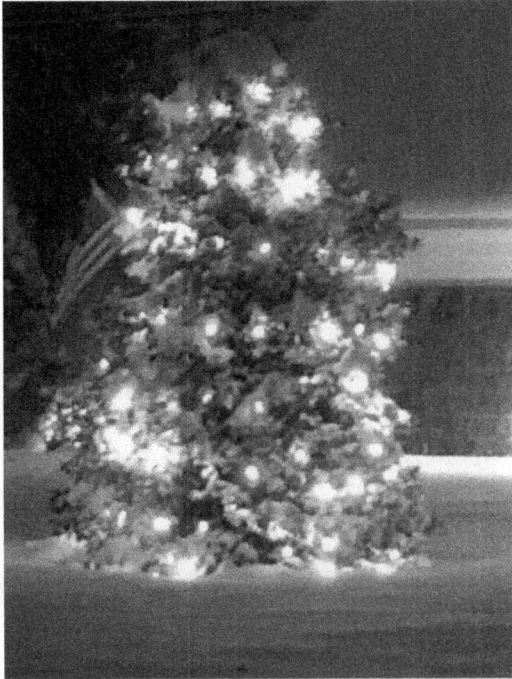

January 11, 2019

Nothing left to take down but the tree! New iPad here! Next week is the big week to start compiling! Found lots of the cards you sent and

hope to have lot of pictures in the book.
Happy New Year to all of you and love and health and peace!

Tomorrow, we travel with Doobert on a leg of the journey to transport a dog named Lucky from a high-kill shelter in Greenville, SC to a new home in Delaware. The journey is undertaken by 9 volunteers, each driving a leg of the trip to get him there in one day. Keep us in your thoughts as we may face some snow and ice but must get him out of the pound where he is!

January 16, 2019

Just a quick update: Despite the snow and ice we made the trip from Richmond to Dale City and back with no problems. Lucky is truly a lucky dog to have so many rescuers to drive a nine-leg journey to safety. Thank you to all of Sandy's family for caring about mom's trip and for the prayers. One more life saved!!!!!

February 1, 2019

Sandy's family. Mom continues the rescue effort and is working to save over 20 German shepherds which are in deplorable conditions. Shenandoah Shepherd Rescue has been trying to help, but the state representative has chosen to ignore this and it is slowly making its way to the Attorneys General if Virginia, but I fear dogs will die unless more voices are added to object to Eric Branscom's decision.

All animal people, please take a moment to read this.
Twenty or more Shepherd dogs are being tethered and in cages without proper shelter on Duncan Chapel Road in Willis, Virginia. The sheriff's office there was advised to ignore this deplorable situation by the representative to the Virginia House of Delegates Eric Branscom. Some of these dogs will die in the cold of this part of Virginia. I have contacted several people including Michelle Welch,

the Assistant Attorney General. We need help getting this public to get these dogs to shelter.

Here is the copy of my email to Eric Branscom. Feel free to copy and post on your page or to your own email message to him. This is urgent. Thank you.

Mr. Branscom,

I am aware that you chose to ignore the advice of our state Attorneys General's office, and in total disregard advised the sheriff's office in Willis, Virginia to ignore the deplorable conditions on Duncan Chapel Road where over 20 dogs are lying in frozen ground and not provided the shelter that the law requires.
It is sad that you have shown a lack of understanding and compassion as a human being and have allowed inhumane treatment of these animals. However, it is my hope that you will choose to reconsider and that all of the public that is now being made aware of this situation will choose to remove you from office if this situation is not remedied.

Should you need assistance with sheltering these dogs or evacuating them from this inhumane situation, I suggest you reach out to Shenandoah German Shepherd Rescue.

Asst. Attorney General is Michelle Welch
Mwelch@oag.state.va.us
Ebranscom@floydcova.org

February 4, 2019

Facebook family. Book began formatting today! Multiple proofreading sessions and deciding what should go where. Excited to have it halfway done!!!! Remembering the cold weather and wonderful blankets and coats. All will be pleased to know that the blankets are used in every rescue drive I make and Annie enjoys hers daily. And, coats are being enjoyed by rescues at Trio Animal Foundation!

We are moving along!! Have the first part of the book with my editor. There are a lot more steps to take with the formatting and putting it all together but we are making good progress. Thanks to all who voted for the cover picture. Am also in process of getting info on specific shelters. Will keep everyone posted on the decision.

We are moving along!! Have the first part of the book with my editor. There are a lot more steps to take with the formatting and putting it all together but we are making good progress. Thanks to all who voted for the cover picture. Am also in process of getting info on specific shelters. Will keep everyone posted on the decision.

After conversations and much thought, the following organizations will be receiving the monies Sandy's Facebook family raised by voting for her book cover and by commenting on the post asking for all of you to send us your favorite choice.

February 24, 2019

We will use Picture Number 1 on the cover.

$100 will go to Southeast German Shepherd Rescue who pulled Sandy from the high kill shelter in North Carolina.

$100 will go to Trio Animal Foundation in Chicago who pulls the worst of the worst abuse and neglect cases off of the streets regardless of breed. They network with veterinarians, behavior specialists, nutrition specialists, and foster throw away dogs and give them new and healthy happy lives.

$150 will go to Best Friends. Best Friends campaign to end all homeless pets by 2022 has resulted in opening two no kill shelters on the east coast, one in New York City and one in Atlanta, GA. Best Friends partners with rescue transports, veterinary hospitals and many shelters around the United States helping them to become shelters with manageable numbers where dogs and cats are literally given a second chance and the medical treatments needed. It is because of my personal experience in volunteering at Best Friends in Utah, that I became active in rescue and animal rights. Being a Virginian and from the hometown of Michael Vick, I first went to Best Friends to volunteer because they had committed to rescue and try to rehabilitate so many of the dogs Michael Vick abused.

Thanks to all of you who participated in this process. The first part of the book is already in my editor's hands and more will follow to her this week.

Blessings and love to all

March 2, 2019

Quick update. Progress on the book continues. Decisions are to be made about where to put pictures and how many. Already have over 100 pages done.

March 4, 2019

It's a wonderful day and we feel joy in sharing this with you! The wheels that Sandy had through the lives and generosity of her Facebook Family have now been donated to help another dog in need. Cutting down a wardrobe moving box to the right size was the big challenge but the wheels are shipped and on the way to leaving another piece of Sandy's legacy.

March 15, 2019

Dear Sandy's Facebook Family

I received this message today from a wonderful mom who is going through degenerative myelopathy with her sweet boxer.

Christine McAuliffe has given me permission to post her message so all of you can know how much your love for Sandy is paying it forward.

From Christine: I'm gonna apologize for the long post, but I'm just as happy as can be right now. My boy Bruce has been down in the back since sometime in August 2018. I have found ways to carry him, get him around, have him still enjoy the company of other doggos, and now that it's been snowy having him enjoy eating his snow. I'd do anything for my soul pup. So, probably about six weeks ago, an incredibly kind person Jenn McEwen gifted me a certificate for Walkin Wheels, but due to unexpected financial obligations, I was unable to purchase Bruce wheels at that time. A couple weeks ago, when funds became available, I was about to make the purchase, when another angel in this group, Diana Blackburn Mahoney, offered me her set of Eddie's Wheels from her dog Sandy. Sadly, Bruce's measurements did not allow us to make the exchange; however, Diana worked hard in an attempt to donate her wheels so that I could in turn get wheels for my boy. I couldn't believe all that she did to facilitate my boy getting wheels.

I am fortunate enough to live about 2 hours away from Eddie's Wheels, so with Diana's help, I made an appointment for Bruce to be measured to see if they had used wheels that would fit him. We were in luck! They had a set that could fit him and hold his chunky butt haha. So, for the last three days, I have put Bruce in his "new-to-you" chariot and taken him for 3 short walks. He's also been able to stand *outside and eat snow (which he LOVES to do). My heart is so full because of these two selfless angels who wanted nothing more than to help a stranger. Here are a couple videos of my boy in his "new" hot rod. With all that being said, the $50 gift certificate that Jenn gave me was not used, and I would like nothing more than to pass it on to another deserving dog mom or dog dad in this group. — with Jenn McEwen and Diana Blackburn Mahoney.*

April 21, 2019

Blessed Day of Saving Grace to all of Sandy's family. Amid the sorrows of Notre Dame and Sri Lanka we all shine the hope that Love Wins.

May 11, 2019

BATMAN4PAWS arrived safely in our driveway from Florida today to hand off four beautiful kitties for an overnight before they journey on to New Jersey tomorrow#batman4paws #doobertrescues #bestfriends #payitforward#nomorehomelesspets #teamtommie

May 16, 2019

Mom is pretty excited today! Dad got a new laptop and now mom can continue her book editing and creating on the laptop and not the iPad with the itsy bits keyboard accessory! Downloaded all the word document to the computer and spent quite some time editing. So much easier on laptop!

August 10, 2019

I know it's been a while. Life gets in the way of our best intentions. Yes, book still in process ...... some editing already done. We never stop remembering Sandy. Her pictures hang prominently in our den, and her photos on our coffee table. As Annie ages, the patience Sandy taught us helps us be more aware of Annie's needs. I am doing volunteer driving for Best Friends and Doobert. Recently we provided overnight accommodation for 4 kitties, and then an overnight for two precious pups who were in the way from Georgia to Canada to their forever homes. My most recent Best Friends run was to drive the very large Best Friends van from Virginia to NYC and back in 24 hours. Took a load of 6 dogs to NYC Best Friends where they were going to foster homes or forever homes. Sandy continues to inspire us. So many of you have adopted or fostered or volunteered with rescues since Sandy's story began and soon I'll be asking everyone to send me a paragraph or sentence or comment about how Sandy inspired you. I believe it needs to be part of the book. Blessings to all.

September 7 2019

To all of Sandy's family, Mom has had to take a hiatus due to a fall off of a ladder. Yes, she was pretty dumb to get on it in the first place. So, considering all the damage it's been hard to update the book; HOWEVER, work will resume next week, and so hope it will be done soon. Dad is taking excellent care of mom and knee replacement is to be determined on the 24th. So, mom couldn't help with the evacuation of animals for Dorian and that was frustrating. Hope everyone this reaches is safe. Remember to send supplies or donations to Best Friends or to your local shelters which are taking in hurricane victims! Thought all of you would like pictures of Sandy.

November 28, 2019

Sending love and best wishes to all of you from Sandy's family. May the blessings of a life well lived be yours, and may your joys come in abundance. Happy Thanksgiving.

December 1, 2019

Hi Sandy's family. Mom got de-railed in September when she fell from a ladder...... her own stubborn fault. As a result she had to have full knee replacement this past Monday and is recuperating (of course, she decorated for Christmas before surgery). The book got delayed with hours of ice and foot propped up. It has to be a New Year resolution. We think of all of you every single day. Sandy's pictures hang prominently in our den, and we continue to spread the message of rescue. It is so heartwarming to know many of you have adopted or volunteered in honor of Sandy's life and how much she was loved. Mom still cries when looking at pictures and the hole Sandy left is just incomprehensible. A bit of really wonderful news! You most probably remember Sandy's cousins, Maggie, Boz, and Pearl and maybe Gabby. Pearl and Gabby were adopted by mom's sister and hubby all because of Sandy. All of them have now crossed the Rainbow Bridge, and now a new rescue is in the works for Mom's sister and hubby! Another miracle! And, as promised but delayed for a lot of reasons that remain concerns, mom and dad rescued another very large big baby named Seamus. He is 96 pounds of pure love and joy. Annie continues to enjoy life when her arthritis isn't a problem. Rest assured you each left indelible prints on our hearts, and we send our love and best wishes for a joyous Christmas season.

December 16, 2019

Three weeks out and mom is walking and doing steps (up only) with the new knee. We did our decorating before surgery, so we send our Christmas Greetings from us to you. How blessed we are by your constant love and friendship.

December 23, 2019

Merry Christmas to all of our friends around the world. May peace be in your hearts, and may you know the joy of loving an animal!

December 31, 2019

We are over the moon happy as we send our love for 2020! One of Sandy's Facebook family members messaged me tonight with details about their new GSD they rescued. They traveled from Tennessee to Alabama to rescue a GSD that needed a home! What wonderful news, and our Sandy is wagging and wagging from heaven! How marvelous that she continues to inspire. What a gift she was!

January 25 2020

Hello Sandy's family. Lotta of things in the works here! Sandy's aunt is getting ready to adopt a Rescue. Mom and dad have been approved as fosters and more stuff to come!

In the meantime, please visit the page called Faye Hope Love. You will see Sandy in this dog's eyes and tell them Sandy sent you! Find it by searching for Shenandoah German Shepherd Rescue.

January 26 2020

Sandy's Facebook Family:

The other two dogs that were found at Faye's address, have now been rescued by Shenandoah Shepherd Rescue. Please read below and share and get in touch with Shenendoah if you can help. Or you can let me know and I will get you in touch with Shenandoah. The need is urgent

From Shenandoah Shepherd Rescue:

The news you have all been waiting for, with another twist...

We got the two remaining GSD's from Faye's property. They are currently at the shelter, and we have a rescue tag on them.

As it turns out, there is one male and one female, and THIS female is pregnant too! She is even further along than Faye and about ready to pop!

Is there anyone in the Houston area who can take on a pregnant female? Potentially the male too? This is news we did not expect, and we do not have a second foster home lined up for another litter!

We need name suggestions and will be posting another wish list to get supplies for more babies. Both pups are suffering from demodectic mange and the female is heartworm positive. They will get better, but they NEED a foster home to do so.

January 25 2020

Posting in honor of the dogs who survived Michael Vick.
As he coaches the Pro Bowl today I hope you will share this to keep making people aware of dog fighting and the subpar humans who participate in it.

February 9 2020

Happy February and Valentine's Day from us to you. So much in the burners right now...... we have been doing some rescue runs for Doobert, have gotten approved for fostering by Shenandoah Shepherd Rescue and awaiting home visit. However, we are holding off a bit because Annie is 14 and terribly weak in her rear legs. We've begun using the yoga mats, as we did with Sandy, so Annie gets traction on the floors. She gets Dasaquin, Gabapentin and Rimadyl to keep her comfortable. She's wagging and happy so we will continue until she is not. Mom has had Annie since she was 6 weeks old. Annie's human sister found her in an equestrian barn at the college when she was a sophomore...... and, of course, mom drove 10 hours to go get Annie and bring her home. Mom and dad dread the inevitability of being without her. As so many of you have experienced the loss of a family pet, our hearts will break again, and we will grieve hard. And we will heal by giving another a home. Mom is afraid of the day coming. She prays the decision will be taken out of her hands but she also knows that won't be the case. We send our love to all of you and ask that you remember Annie and us in your thoughts and prayers in these days. If there are prayers needed by any of you please know they are available for the asking.

February 10 2020

We visited our wonderful veterinary office, Sycamore Veterinary, in Midlothian, Virginia today. Annie will now be on gabapentin routinely to see if that helps, and having acupuncture to address her sore back. She's better today but the days of doing stairs are gone. We will do all we can to ensure her quality of life and her happiness. Thanks to each one of you for the kind and loving messages you sent. Mom's spirits were lifted, and a good night's sleep followed!

February 13 2020

Mom sees so many posts about people who are dealing with losing their fur babies. It is so heartbreaking and all too familiar. Sandy and Buddy left such big holes in our family and now we face the days when Annie can no longer walk. We pray for strength and courage and peace for all of you and for us.

February 16 2020

Just a quick update:

Mom worked on the book for hours this weekend.
Annie has lost use of both back legs and we have an appointment for acupuncture tomorrow as well as another vet visit. We are very concerned that this is DM and having to breathe deeply about the possibility of doing it all over again.

February 17 2020

Not good news about Annie but reminding myself every other minute how lucky we have been to have her for so long. Her problem is neurological and due to her age we will keep her comfortable as long as she is happy. We are using Sandy's Help Em Up Harness which adjusted to fit Annie. She's still able to go out with assistance to use the potty so Sandy trained us well. Thank you for all the prayers and healing blessings. Each one brings a bit of peace to us, and we are blessed by so many of you who have been with us all these years. Most of you have walked the path we are on so we know we are all part of life's journey. Love to all.

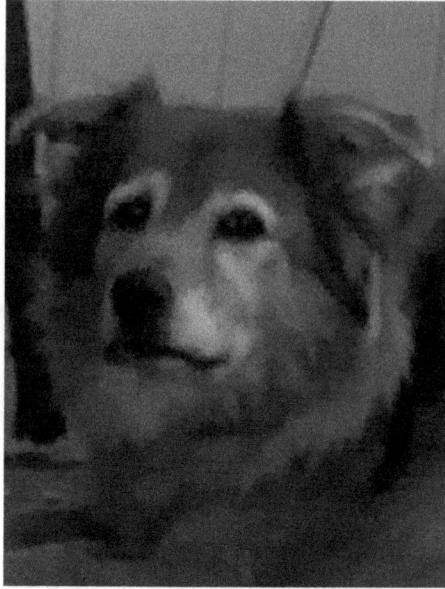

February 22 2020

Thank you to all for the thoughts and prayers. We are asking God for strength and wisdom. Letting go and knowing it is close to time. We keep all of you who have gone or will go through this in our heart and I draw strength from knowing all of you truly understand.

February 25 2020

Aching bones
Bright eyes
Dangling feet
Wagging tail
Soft blankets and harness
Lord help my mom and dad.
Aching hearts

Leaking eyes
And strength for all of us.

Broken hearts
Wrenching guts
Pain unavoidable
Walking through devastation
To love always and pass to another.

The price we pay
The deal we make
The path we choose
Ours to make a difference.

Sincere thanks to all for the expressions of sympathy and kindness to us.

March 1 2020

Facebook family, we want to read and absorb every loving comment you made about Annie. Trouble is, mom can only read a few without the tears blurring her eyes so just know as we "like" your comments and best wishes and prayers, we will be slow to respond but will get better day after day. Just to lift some spirits, we are already pursuing adopting as well as fostering. We know we are meant to do this and we will keep you posted on this as we go. For those of you who have loved a four-legged family member we send our heartfelt thanks for you loving them. For those with pets who still enjoy this life we urge you to love them every minute, and for those whose pets are suffering and having to make hard decisions, we keep you in our prayers.

March 10, 2020

The flowers from a dear friend sent after Annie's journey onward are still blooming. Annie began to lose all the strength in her back legs very rapidly. Within two weeks, she went from walking on all four feet to dragging her legs and attempting to scoot across the floor. Within the last three days of her life with us she lost control of her bladder and bowels and life was stressing her. Mom called and made THE appointment with our trusted veterinary practice, Sycamore Veterinary Animal Clinic. The day arrived. Mom and Dad worked hard to not let her see us fall to pieces. Their stomachs were in knots, their sorrow stuffed down inside while we showered her with a steak and treats and chocolate ......yes, the chocolate that is poison for dogs and that she had never had but always wanted...oh, except for that one time she slyly ate a candy bowl full of Hershey's kisses many years ago. Dad sat beside her, and mom got on the floor beside her. Mom told her what a good girl she was and that everything would be ok. She is ok. We are working on it. Thanks to all for the wonderful messages and comments. Sandy and Annie and Buddy are alive and well in our hearts.

The Rescue Continues

We thought all of you could use some good news and feel the joy with us! Welcome adopted puppy (8 weeks old and 8 pounds) currently called Juniper. The Mahoney family passes on Sandy's legacy of adoption!

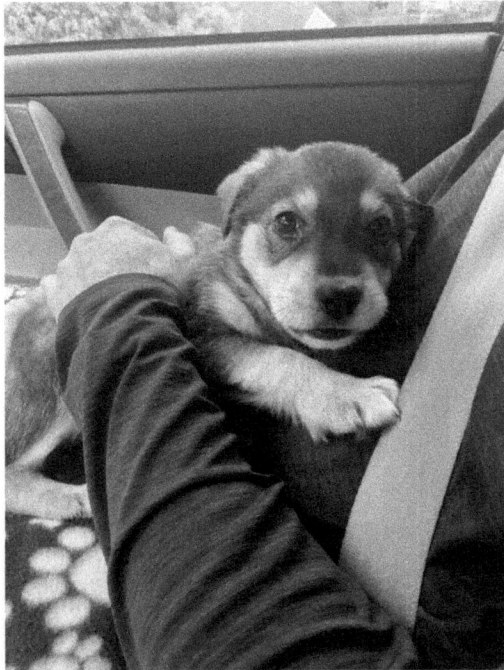

Juniper at 8 weeks

March 16, 2020

Sending all of our Facebook family our prayers for your health and safety. Thought this picture might make you smile. She hates that new collar; no, she doesn't have fleas but is trying to scratch the collar off.

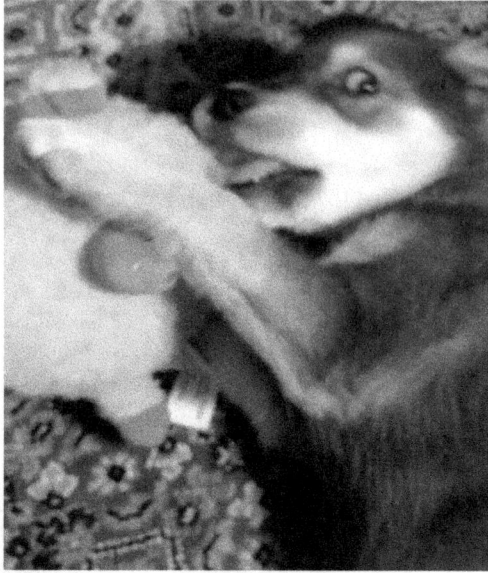

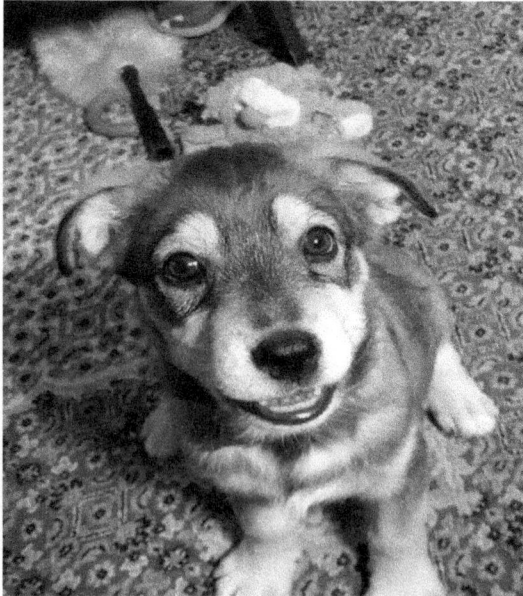

Juniper at 7 weeks

March 23 2020

Thinking of all of you all over the world. We are well and have been staying at home for the past week. Our rescued Labrador and our baby girl named Juniper. Too cute and hope to make you smile. Such a strange time, and mom is even more grateful for all of you!

April 7 2020

Hoping with all our hearts that all of our Facebook family is ok and not taking chances. To any of you who are having to work or attend to the sick, you are true heroes.
If any of you are lonely and just need to chat, message us on this page! We'd love to hear from you!

Our new addition is growing like a weed and coming along with the potty training. The sweet dog, Faye, whom we are following on Shenandoah Shepherd Rescue, became a foster failure and was adopted into her foster family. A happy note for another point of grace. I'm adding pictures for your enjoyment. Praying for all of you.

April 8 2020

Today is National Dogfighting Day which brings attention to the horror of dog fighting. Virginia is not yet clean and rid of dog fighting. If you see something, say something. We have a horrible dog situation in Southwest Virginia, and the local law enforcement turns a blind eye.

April 20, 2020

Sandy's blanket is being put to good use by a full-tummy Juniper. She weighed 17 pounds on Tuesday; a 12 1/2 weeks. She keeps us busy but *sleeps in her kennel all night with no problem. Planting flowers is a challenge because she wants to dig right where I am digging. This week and the next few are critical to her socialization, so we've been to Home Depot with masks and gloves and walked around the neighborhood. We hope all of you are well and that all of you are being careful. It's so easy to feel stressed by this sheltering in place. Days seem to run together. Mom is grateful for being able to work in the yard, but we all miss our family and friends. Juniper and Cash are doing great and she has developed quite an insistent little whine when he has something she wants. Hope you enjoy the video! Love to all!*

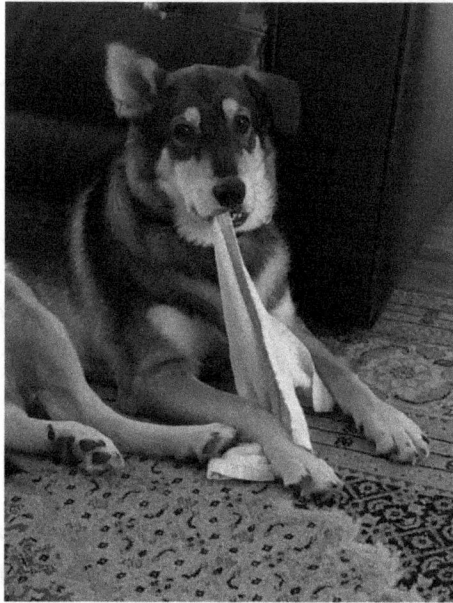

Juniper at 3 years old

July 22, 2020

Hello all dear friends. I am finally editing the book. I am to the point now of adding pictures, then on to press!
In reading again and again her story, I had avoided what was written

in the final days. I have just re-read the tributes and prayers for her and, in particular, the parting prayer by Carol Albrecht. So, my editing is finished for the day because the tears still come.

August 16, 2020

Hello all of you wonderful people who loved Sandy so much. I've been going through a lot of pictures and found myself deeply emotional over the ones of Sandy. I really am going to finish the book. I've been delayed because I started volunteering for Shenandoah Shepherd Rescue and am now reviewing applications for the rescues and doing home visits to ensure each dog goes to a home where it will thrive. During Covid, the application interviews have had to be done on Zoom, as have many of the home visits and there is an endless stream of dogs we are rescuing out of Texas. In south Texas, it is a status symbol to have a German Shepherd or a Belgian Malinois. They are bred for money and when a young dog needs training so badly, as these dogs require, people say they are too much trouble or too stubborn or misbehaving or too big etc. so, they take these dogs and drop them in the streets, the desert, sometimes tie them up and leave them. They take momma dogs and puppies and drop them off in remote areas, sometimes with nothing and sometimes in a cooler. It is horrible. And the stream of dogs never stops. It has consumed much of my time, and on top of that, I'm chairwoman of the committee for my high school's 50th reunion. Covid has complicated this, as I'm sure it has complicated life for each of you. We all yearn for some sense of normalcy, and just when we think we are seeing the end of the tunnel, here we go again.

My husband and I have been vaccinated and will be eligible for the booster soon. I urge all of you dear ones to get vaccinated! I'm so concerned about all of the variants that will occur unless all of us put up barriers to this virus being passed around. Our year and a half old

GSD/Husky rescue is named Juniper. She is adorable and has all the stubborn hardheaded nature of both breeds. She's very smart and very vocal. You may also remember that when Sandy was alive, we had a gorgeous black Lab next door to us named Cash. He and his human mom and his human brother and sister were abandoned by their dad. The sister is non-verbal autistic, and Cash had been in the way of her involuntary movements and fallen several times, so we adopted him. He is 12 years old and an absolutely perfect dog! Juniper loves him, and he's been good about teaching her limits on being a pest!

I'll be back to work on the book after October 1. Please, all of you, stay safe, be careful and get vaccinated. I'll be in touch more often. Sending all of you heartfelt love and appreciation.

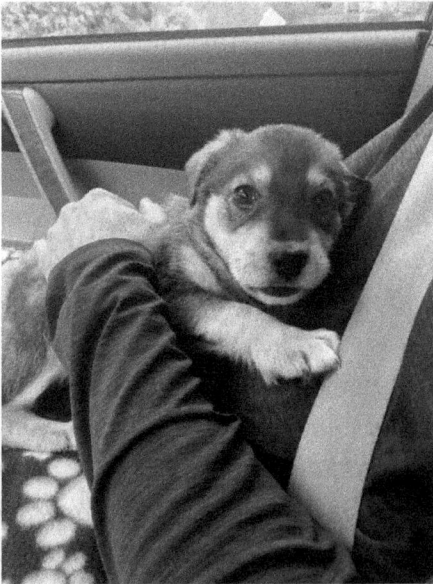

Juniper at 8 weeks

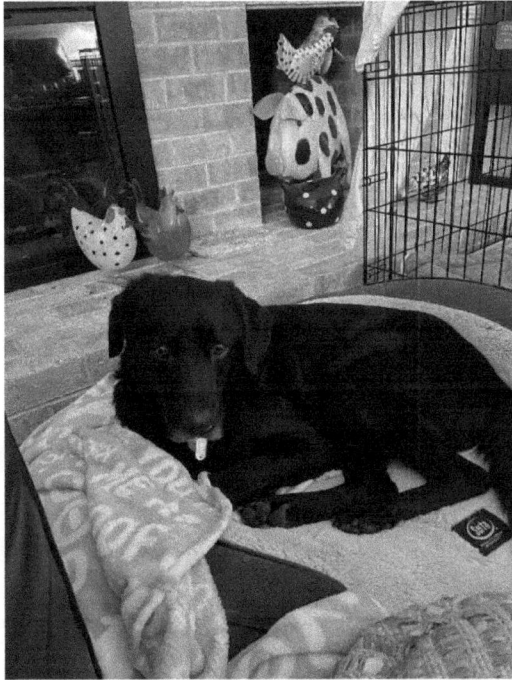

Rocky at 4 years

Note: And, lo and behold, it is 2022, and the story is now complete. I am so thankful for each person who followed Sandy and for the gracious and generous gifts that enabled her to have the best life possible while with us. We now have two rescues, one who is a Husky Shepherd mix named Juniper, and a black Labrador Retriever who is named Rocky. They are the beneficiaries of so much we learned about adopting.

...And I realize that I had no idea this book would be 400-some-odd pages.

My wish in writing this book is to continue to make humans aware of their duty to the creatures over which they have dominion. I have been blessed knowing so many of Sandy's Facebook family have gone on to adopt, to volunteer, to foster, and speak out for these amazing and resilient creatures. I thank each of you who followed her in her journey and shared the good days and the bad days with us. I thank you for your words, your prayers, your thoughts and deeds, and for a feeling of everlasting friendship. May you always travel on your journey knowing you are appreciated, that you did, can and do make a difference to animals in need, inspiring others to do it also.

Blessings on you always.

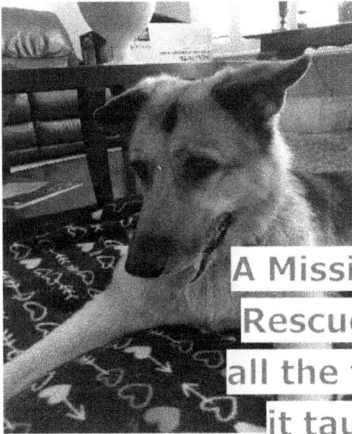

A Mission To
Rescue and
all the things
it taught

When Diana Blackburn Mahoney got a late-night call that rescue was needed, she and her husband dove right in, not knowing anything about the dog in danger of euthanization, but determined she should have a chance. The efforts of a woman named Sandy to keep her from being euthanized resulted in a call to Southeast German Shepherd Rescue. A kind woman named Lorraine called Diana and asked for help. The result was the journey of a lifetime, a lesson for the ages, and witnessing the indomitable spirit of one German Shepherd they named Sandy.

Diana and her husband, Michael, continue to rescue and provide a home for animals who need them. Diana shares their experience through the voice of Sandy, at times heartbreaking and at times quite humorous. Diana's journal of Sandy's experience was kept on social media, where Sandy eventually had over 16,000 followers.

This incredibly inspiring and touching piece of literary work is not only for dog lovers who support rescue but for anyone touched by the spirit of an animal who forgives so freely.

www.ingramcontent.com/pod-product-compliance
Lightning Source LLC
Chambersburg PA
CBHW062112020426
42335CB00013B/933